Oxford Guide to CBT for People with Cancer

Oxford Guide to CBT for People with Cancer

SECOND EDITION

Stirling Moorey, MB BS, BSc, FRCPsych

Consultant Medical Psychotherapist, South London and Maudsley NHS Foundation Trust, and Honorary Senior Lecturer, Institute of Psychiatry, London, UK

Steven Greer, MD, FRCPsych, FRANZCP

Consultant Psychiatrist, St Raphael's Hospice, Sutton, Surrey, and Emeritus Reader in Psychological Medicine, Institute of Cancer Research, University of London, London, UK

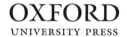

OXFORD
UNIVERSITY PRESS

OXFORD
UNIVERSITY PRESS

Great Clarendon Street, Oxford ox2 6dp

Oxford University Press is a department of the University of Oxford.
It furthers the University's objective of excellence in research, scholarship,
and education by publishing worldwide in

Oxford New York

Auckland Cape Town Dar es Salaam Hong Kong Karachi
Kuala Lumpur Madrid Melbourne Mexico City Nairobi
New Delhi Shanghai Taipei Toronto

With offices in

Argentina Austria Brazil Chile Czech Republic France Greece
Guatemala Hungary Italy Japan Poland Portugal Singapore
South Korea Switzerland Thailand Turkey Ukraine Vietnam

Oxford is a registered trade mark of Oxford University Press
in the UK and in certain other countries

Published in the United States
by Oxford University Press Inc., New York

British Library Cataloguing in Publication Data
Data available

Library of Congress Cataloging in Publication Data
Data available

Typeset in Minion by Cenveo, Bangalore, India
Printed and bound by CPI Group (UK) Ltd,
Croydon, CR0 4YY

ISBN 978–0–19–960580–4

10 9 8 7 6 5 4 3 2 1

Foreword

Like many others, I view my time on airplanes as an opportunity to catch up on reading. No e-mail, no phone calls, no conversations with colleagues, friends, and family; just a stretch of time that is all mine. However, my expectations often prove to be overly optimistic, especially when my reading material contains the words 'stress' or 'coping' in the title. In such instances, my seatmate is likely to glance at whatever it is that I'm reading and then, leaning towards me and speaking in a slightly conspiratorial voice, either offer to tell me about the stress in his or her life or ask me to share the secrets of successful coping, of course, to be summarized in just a few words. Usually I listen to the stories about stress not just to be polite, but because I find such stories interesting and often quite moving. But when I am asked to share the secrets of successful coping, I reveal that I am a psychologist who does research and not a psychologist who sees patients. Usually that response precipitates an immediate loss of interest and I am left, once again, with the promise of uninterrupted time in which to work.

My seatmates probably assume that as a researcher I am good with data but ill-equipped to speak about the meaning of the data in relation to helping people get through difficult days. This assumption is in fact deeply embedded in the cultures of the social and behavioral sciences on the one hand and clinical practice on the other. Historically, the two cultures have evolved separately; they have spoken different languages and have had different objectives. The social and behavioral sciences, for example, have focused on explaining and even predicting behavior, while clinical practice has focused on diagnosing and treating adjustment problems and mental illness. In recent years, however, each discipline is finding reasons to reach across the chasm to the other, to build bridges that permit flow of knowledge and promote multidisciplinary collaboration.

One concept in particular has played a key role in bridging the chasm: stress. On the clinical side, stress is recognized as a cause of behaviors such as smoking, drinking, overeating, and use of illegal drugs that can cause disease and even death. The study of such behaviors has resided primarily with the social and behavioral scientists, which means clinicians need to reach out to the researchers. On the other hand, social and behavioral scientists are increasingly interested in how psychological processes associated with stress adversely affect organ systems and eventuate in disease. Advances in technology are making it possible to pursue such questions, so now the researchers want to connect with clinicians and their patient populations.

Stirling Moorey and Steven Greer illustrate the bridge-building process. Moorey and Greer developed Adjuvant Psychological Therapy to support the well-being of patients with cancer. Then they conducted clinical research to determine, among other objectives, the effects of their treatment and the replicability of their earlier findings. At the same time, and possibly influenced by Moorey and Greer's pioneering work, others developed and tested variations of cognitive behavioral therapy designed for cancer patients. By the late 1990s, sufficient numbers of studies had been conducted to allow a meta analysis. The benefits as well as the limitations of cognitive behavioral treatments in general and Adjuvant Psychological Therapy in particular were identified.

The current edition shows a deepened understanding of the patient populations for which cognitive behavioral treatments can be most effective and for issues faced by diverse patient groups. The authors' experience also informs the discussion of how the therapist should engage the patient at various phases not only of illness, but also of therapy such as entry, mid-way and exit.

At the time of Moorey and Greer's first edition, the field of psycho-oncology was in its infancy. The dramatic expansion in the intervening decades includes the development of evidence-based treatments to support the quality of life and well-being of patients with chronic illness or the prospect of imminent death. The work of Moorey and Greer has continued throughout this period of expansion. The process through which they have developed their treatment, using their first-hand experience with cancer patients tempered with their own research as well as the research of others, illustrates the way research and practice can be mutually beneficial.

As for my airplane conundrum, next time I will place Moorey and Greer's book on top of my reading pile, thereby eliciting interest primarily from those with a specific interest in cancer. I will offer my seatmate the Moorey and Greer book for the duration of the flight. This act has two purposes: it will provide the opportunity for my seatmate to begin learning about the complexity of coping with cancer while also protecting my precious airplane reading time.

Susan Folkman
San Mateo, CA
July, 2011

As no two persons are alike in health, so no two are alike in disease: and no diagnosis is complete or exact which does not include an estimate of the character or constitution of the patient … for to treat a sick man rightly requires diagnosis not only of the disease but the manner and degrees in which its supposed essential characteristics are modified by his personal qualities, by the inheritances that converge in him, by the changes wrought in him by the conditions of his past life, and many things besides.

James Paget (1885)
Address to Abernethian Society

Preface

When the first incarnation of this book was published in 1989, Professor Tim McElwain, one of Britain's most eminent oncologists, wrote in the Preface:

> 'Of course what we have here is very much a work in progress, and clearly there will be more to be done to refine, augment and validate the treatments advocated; but I feel certain that this important book will be of immediate value to everyone concerned with the management of cancer patients.'

In the 20 years since this was written, cognitive therapy has established itself as the psychological therapy with the strongest evidence base, and psycho-oncology has firmly established itself as a branch of health psychology. Our own work has moved from the area of early-stage, curable cancer to the field of palliative care, and this change is reflected in an expansion of the chapter on advanced disease and a new chapter on working with grief. Interventions in psycho-oncology are becoming more sophisticated, and we now give more attention to the adaptation of cognitive behaviour therapy (CBT) for specific cancer problems and symptoms. CBT has also increased its understanding of psychological processes such as selective attention, safety behaviours, and the role of worry and rumination in maintaining disorders, and we have incorporated some of these insights into our treatment. Readers of the previous editions have valued the clarity of the text, and we have not sought to change it substantially, but rather to update it in the light of recent research and clinical developments. We have retained the two-part structure. Part One describes some of the key clinical, theoretical, and empirical aspects of the psychology of cancer. It begins with an account of the experiences of people with cancer and the common emotional reactions to the disease. In Chapter 2 these reactions are put into a cognitive behavioural context, with an updated cognitive model of adjustment to cancer. Chapters 3 and 4 review the evidence both for the effectiveness of cognitive behavioural interventions in people with cancer, and for the impact of therapy on the disease process itself. Part Two is a description of our version of CBT for people with cancer, namely adjuvant psychological therapy. It begins with an overview of adjuvant psychological therapy in Chapter 5, followed by a description of the structure and nature of the therapeutic relationship in Chapter 6. Chapters 7, 8, and 9 present the basic emotional, behavioural, and cognitive techniques that are used in therapy. These remain unchanged from the last edition, except for some updating of Chapter 7 in the light of more recent thoughts on experiential avoidance. We have separated techniques for working with anxiety and depression (described in Chapter 10) from techniques for other common problems (covered in Chapter 11). This has allowed an expansion of the section on managing anxiety, to include more material on worry and panic. Chapter 11 now contains more detailed information on how to work with insomnia, fatigue, pain, and nausea, in addition to anger. Chapter 12 gives more guidance on how to create a developmental conceptualization and how to work with underlying beliefs. Chapter 13 describes how partners can be included in the therapy session. Chapter 14 addresses the special application of CBT to people with advanced disease or terminal illness. This is a challenging and rewarding area of work, which has traditionally been more the preserve of humanistic and supportive therapies. In Chapter 15 we describe the application of cognitive behavioural techniques to grief reactions and, as in the previous edition, we conclude with a chapter on working with groups. We hope that this book continues to be easily readable (i.e. as free from jargon as possible), informative and, above all, of immediate practical use for professionals who are involved in the clinical care of patients with cancer. It should be of interest to nurses and oncologists who wish to learn how to apply a problem-focused approach to their patients' psychological concerns, and should also be a useful resource for psychologists, psychiatrists, and other mental health professionals working in medical settings.

We would like to thank Kathy Burn and Lyn Snowden for the clinical discussions that have formed the basis for some of the new material in the book, as well as Magda Moorey for helpful comments on an earlier draft, and Carol Sells for her unfailing support during the preparation of this book. As always it is our patients who have taught us most, and we remain deeply indebted to them.

Stirling Moorey
Steven Greer

Contents

List of abbreviations

APT	Adjuvant psychological therapy
BDI	Beck Depression Inventory
BPP	Biobehavioral Pain Profile
CBT	Cognitive behavioural therapy
CCQ	Cancer Coping Questionnaire
CTFARS	Cognitive Therapy First Aid Rating Scale
DTR	Dysfunctional Thought Record
HADS	Hospital Anxiety and Depression Scale
HDRS	Hamilton Depression Rating Scale
MACS	Mental Adjustment to Cancer Scale
MASCC	Multinational Association of Supportive Care in Cancer
NICE	National Institute for Health and Clinical Excellence
PAIS	Psychosocial Adjustment to Illness Scale
POMS	Profile of Mood States
RSCL	Rotterdam Symptom Checklist
STAI	State-Trait Anxiety Inventory

Part One

The Psychology of Cancer

Chapter 1

What people with cancer feel

John was a 26-year-old bricklayer who led an active life, dividing his time between his girlfriend, his mates, and football, although not necessarily in that order. He was a strong healthy man who enjoyed life and who had no previous history of serious physical or psychiatric illness. One day while they were making love his girlfriend noticed that his left testicle was swollen. She persuaded him to see his doctor, who referred him to an oncologist. John was found to have testicular cancer. That same evening, after writing suicide notes to his mother and his girlfriend, he killed himself with a massive drug overdose. The tragedy of this man's death was compounded by the fact that testicular germ-cell tumours in young adult men are highly curable (Horwich, 1995). Fortunately, such tragic cases are rare, but they illustrate the high level of emotional distress that cancer can evoke.

The correct diagnosis is needed

There can be little doubt that a diagnosis of cancer evokes in most people a dread which exceeds that of other diseases which carry equally serious or worse prognoses (McIntosh, 1974). Despite well-publicized progress in treatment, for many people the word 'cancer' suggests a wild, uncontrollable proliferation of cells destroying the body and leading to a slow, painful death. Not surprisingly, therefore, doctors have until relatively recently shielded patients from learning the diagnosis. How do patients feel about this? To appreciate how they may feel, imagine that you are a patient who has developed cancer. Your doctor, believing that you cannot cope with the truth, refuses to give you the correct diagnosis and instead fobs you off with euphemisms. Your partner or close relative is told that you have cancer, and is advised on no account to reveal the diagnosis to you, but rather to maintain a cheerful facade in front of you. Meanwhile, your symptoms grow worse, you begin to suspect that you might have cancer, but neither your doctor nor your nearest and dearest will tell you the truth. You are told that you require an operation. You are admitted to a general surgical ward. There you become uneasily aware of an all-too-common practice; on ward rounds, the surgical team stand at the foot of your bed and discuss your case in low whispers, and you notice that they do not do this when dealing with other patients on the ward. Feeling isolated and increasingly anxious and helpless, you undergo major surgery. In this climate of fear and uncertainty it is highly likely that you will experience intense emotional distress.

Experiences of this kind were common in the 1950s and 1960s. An American survey at that time reported that as many as 90% of doctors did not reveal the diagnosis of cancer to their patients (Oken, 1961). This was also conventional practice in Britain. Doubtless, doctors who shielded patients from this dreaded diagnosis acted with the best intentions. But were they right to do so? In what was a daring British pioneer study, given the climate of opinion at that time, a series of patients with cancer attending hospital for radiotherapy were told the diagnosis, and their reactions were assessed 1 to 4 weeks later (Aitken-Swan and Easson, 1959). The results were instructive. They revealed that 66% of the patients approved of the fact that they had been told they had cancer, only 7% disapproved, and, interestingly, 19% denied that they had been told (the reactions of the remaining 7% could not be ascertained). This salient finding, that a large majority of patients with cancer wanted to be informed of the diagnosis, began to bring about a change in medical attitudes and clinical practice. Although the practice of not revealing a cancer diagnosis to patients persists to this day in Southern and Eastern Europe, disclosure of the diagnosis is now common practice in Western Europe, North America and Australia (Holland and Marchini, 1998). However, the change in medical attitudes is not confined to disclosing the diagnosis, welcome though that is. There has been a sea change from the paternalistic attitude adopted by many surgeons towards a more evenly balanced professional relationship in which the patient is fully informed about their disease, or rather as informed as they wish to be, and is invited to take part in decisions regarding treatment. At least this is what is supposed to have happened. In reality, the change has been slow in coming, and has been patchy throughout the UK. In the following account, a patient describes her experience (in 1998) to one of the authors:

> I started getting pains in my stomach and I thought it was just indigestion. Then I started getting constipated, but sometimes diarrhoea as well. I began to go off my food. My husband made me go to the doctor, who sent me to the hospital. They did some very unpleasant tests but never told me what it was. The surgeon asked me to wait outside while he spoke to my husband. All I could get out of either of them was that there was a bit of my bowel which wasn't right, and I had to have an operation and then some drugs afterwards. I began to worry that it was something serious – I couldn't get it out of my mind.
>
> I thought 'Could it be the big C?', but when I finally plucked up the courage to ask, the surgeon just said 'You mustn't worry yourself – it's a bit of bowel that isn't working properly, and when we take it out you should be all right.' After the operation,

I was given drugs which made me feel sick all the time. I lost my appetite, got more and more pain, and just felt awful. I worried the whole time and used to cry a lot when on my own. My husband and daughter used to try to cheer me up by saying 'You'll get better soon', but after a while I didn't believe them any more. I got more and more frightened and shaky and couldn't eat. I felt completely alone, and the worst part was not knowing, not being able to talk to anyone. It's funny, now that you have told me what's really wrong with me, I somehow feel stronger in myself. I know it's very serious and I'm still frightened, but not like before. I honestly feel better for knowing the truth. It's such a relief to be able to talk about it.

Anxiety and depression

Giving the patient the diagnosis is not enough on its own. The traumatic impact of a cancer diagnosis requires close attention to the patient's emotional needs. However, since the advent of high-technology medicine and increasingly narrow specialization, this important aspect of medical care has become relatively neglected. What patients feel when their emotional needs are ignored can be illustrated by their own comments.

The following comment was made by a physician suffering from lymphoma:

> Today's oncologists need to be encouraged to derive feelings of self-esteem and career satisfaction from improving the quality as well as the quantity of the patient's existence. By addressing the emotional problems associated with chemotherapy, they can diminish their patient's feelings of abandonment and rage and prevent the despair which patients suffer.

(Cohn, 1982)

A patient with Hodgkin's disease commented as follows:

> … my experiences have taught me that adjusting to life with Hodgkin's disease has as much to do with emotional attitudes and communication as with physical states… while doctors still inquire 'How do you feel?', it seems to me that increasing reliance upon high-technology diagnostic equipment has led to a decreasing emphasis on the importance of my reporting my body state. I came to resent this.

(Cooper, 1982)

Faced with a diagnosis of cancer, most people react initially with numbed shock and disbelief, followed by anxiety, anger, and depression. In the majority of cases, this stress reaction subsides within a few weeks as they learn, painfully and slowly, to come to terms with their disease. Patients can be helped to make this adjustment by their doctor's sensitive sympathetic counsel, and by the emotional support of family and close friends. However, a substantial minority go on to develop persistent psychological disorders. In our study of 1260 patients with various cancers attending the Royal Marsden Hospital, who were screened psychologically 4 to 12 weeks after an initial diagnosis of cancer,

23% were found to have clinically significant anxiety (15%) or depression (8%) (Greer et al, 1992). In addition, some patients who cope well with the initial diagnosis are psychologically overwhelmed subsequently by the news that their cancers have recurred or spread. At the most conservative estimate, 25–30% of patients suffer from cancer-related psychological disorders. If left untreated, these disorders may persist for years even in the absence of any evidence of disease (Morris et al, 1977; Fobair et al, 1986; Irvine et al, 1991; Kornblith et al, 1992). For example, a prospective study of an unselected series of patients with breast, lung, and colorectal cancers revealed that there was no improvement in psychological adaptation over time. In fact, a significant decline in mental health scores between baseline assessment and 1–2 years after diagnosis was found (Ell et al, 1989). More recent studies have confirmed these findings. A study which followed 222 women with breast cancer over 5 years found rates of anxiety and depression of 33% at diagnosis, 15% at 1 year (when most women had been successfully treated and were disease free), and 45% when there was a recurrence (Burgess et al, 2005).

In the early stages it may be treatment which causes most distress, rather than the effects of the disease itself. Surgery is often tolerated as a 'necessary evil' because it is seen as a treatment that will root the cancer out, but subsequent chemotherapy and radiotherapy can be more difficult to deal with, particularly if they are given as prophylactic treatments to patients who are otherwise feeling well. Mastectomy has been shown to be associated with high levels of anxiety and depression (Morris et al, 1977; Maguire et al, 1978; Grandi et al, 1987), with up to a quarter of women remaining depressed 1 year after the operation. However, there seems to be a similar incidence of psychological morbidity in lumpectomy patients and mastectomy patients (Fallowfield et al, 1986; van Heeringen et al, 1990). Around 25–50% of colostomy patients experience psychological problems (Devlin et al, 1971; Wirsching et al, 1975; Eardley et al, 1976). High rates of depression and work-related problems were found in people who had undergone laryngectomy (Barton, 1965; Drummond, 1967).

Radiotherapy commonly causes nausea and fatigue (Peck, 1972; Greenberg et al, 1992), and it may sometimes be difficult to distinguish these symptoms from the lethargy that is experienced in depressive reactions. Agitation, withdrawal, non-engagement with treatment, and unrealistic expectations of treatment have been cited as predictors of poor outcome in radiotherapy (Schmale et al, 1982). In a recent study, Montgomery et al (1999) reported that 30% of patients who were receiving radiotherapy reached caseness for adjustment disorder and/or anxiety/depression. Chemotherapy is also associated with high levels of anxiety and depression – for example, 40% of patients in a study by Middelboe et al (1995). The incidence of psychological problems may be lower when chemotherapy is given to produce symptomatic improvement, as for example in lung cancer (Hughes, 1985), than when it is given as a prophylactic treatment.

Systematic studies of psychological morbidity among patients with cancer provide useful statistical data. However, nothing can convey what these patients really feel as vividly as their own descriptions. A 57-year-old man described how he felt upon learning that he had developed lung cancer:

> At first I couldn't take it in, I didn't believe it.... I went all numb, then I thought perhaps the doctors have made a mistake, you read about it all the time. But deep down I knew I had cancer... I was very, very scared at first, then I felt very low. I went into my shell, didn't want to see anyone; I couldn't tell my wife how I felt, I still can't.

A 36-year-old woman had undergone a mastectomy followed by chemotherapy, and was put on long-term tamoxifen. After 18 months she was found to have a metastatic deposit in her sternum:

> It's hard to describe what I feel; fear, of course, utter misery, helplessness. It was bad enough the first time.... I went through all that chemo and had my breast off and now it turns out it was all for nothing.

Disturbed relationships

In addition to anxiety and depressive states, patients have reported other difficulties in their lives, particularly sexual dysfunction (e.g. Morris et al, 1977; Andersen, 1986; Northouse et al, 1998). The effect of cancer on marital and other intimate relationships will depend in part on the previous quality of these relationships. The impact of cancer often exacerbates pre-existing problems. For instance, men who perceive illness as weakness, and who have a need to control others or avoid confrontation find it harder to cope with their partner's breast cancer, and this impairs marital interactions (Carter et al, 1993). On the other hand, previously close relationships are rarely damaged, and may become even closer as the threat of cancer to life makes both partners realize how important they are to each other (Morris et al, 1977; Zucchero, 1998). Good marital relationships can buffer the stress of cancer, and are associated with less psychological distress in the patient (Rodrigue and Park, 1996).

Less well recognized than marital problems, but no less important, is the effect that breast cancer may have on the mother–daughter relationship (Lichtman and Taylor, 1986; Wellisch et al, 1992; Zahlis and Lewis, 1998). Mothers of adolescent daughters in particular have reported dramatic rejecting responses. In the words of one mother with breast cancer:

My daughter went out of her way to make it harder for me. She would come in and she would make a mess in the kitchen, knowing that I couldn't clean it up. One night, she simply took off and left a note saying that she had to get out of the house. We didn't know where she was, and I was completely hysterical.

(Lichtman et al, 1985)

Sexual dysfunction

A common but insufficiently recognized complication of cancer is sexual dysfunction (Schover, 1998). Sexual problems can be a consequence of cancer-related anxiety and depression, or may result from psychological and physical damage following certain treatments, such as disfiguring surgery, ostomies, surgical nerve damage, radical pelvic irradiation, and the side-effects of chemotherapy and hormone treatment.

A 64-year-old man with a colostomy following surgery for cancer of the colon was referred for depression:

To tell you the truth, doctor, I've been depressed since I had the operation last February [8 months ago]. Don't think I'm not grateful to the surgeon, he did what he had to do, he cut out the cancer. It's just that I hate this bag so much; I can't get used to it. I'm frightened it will leak or smell. I don't go anywhere or do anything. [How does your wife feel about it?] Well... she's very good about it... but, to tell you the truth... it's hard to say this, but I'm not a man any more. That's made me feel worse than anything.... I'm really sad about that. My wife says it doesn't matter, but I know it does. She's a lot younger than me; we've always had a good sex life. Now it's all gone (he has tears in his eyes).

A 42-year-old woman described her feelings one year after mastectomy:

I'm not a complete woman any more. My partner has tried to reassure me, but I feel so unattractive.... I look horrible; I looked at the scar once and quickly turned away from the mirror. I've never looked at my chest since. When I have a bath I cover my top half up. I've never let Jim see me naked, and we haven't made love since the operation. It's put a great strain on our relationship.... Jim says he loves me and wants me, but I couldn't bear him to touch me there and see how ugly I am now.

In the literature on the complications of cancer treatments, with rare exceptions sexual functioning is either completely ignored or given short shrift. It would appear that many clinicians consider it inappropriate to discuss sexual matters in the context of cancer, and many older patients in particular are too embarrassed to mention this topic. Such embarrassment can be easily overcome if clinicians routinely enquire about sexual function as part of their assessment of the quality of life of patients. It is important to obtain information about sexual dysfunction for two reasons. First, such information will encourage the development of nerve-sparing surgical procedures – for example, replacing abdomino-perineal resection with low sphincter-saving resection for rectal cancer (Williams and Johnston, 1983). Secondly, effective treatment for sexual dysfunction is now possible in many cases (see Chapter 11).

Acute confusional states

So far we have described what are essentially chronic psychological disorders among patients with cancer. Acute disturbances, although less common, may also arise in the form of confusional states. Patients become restless, suspicious, noisy, angry, and confused, with impaired concentration, memory, and orientation for time and place. Their mood is usually abnormal, ranging from depression to euphoria. Acute confusional states are often worse at night. Opioid analgesics are the commonest cause. Other causes include steroids, certain chemotherapeutic agents (e.g. cis-platinum, interferon, and vincristine), primary or secondary cerebral tumours, and encephalopathy due to metabolic disturbances such as hypercalcaemia and electrolyte imbalance, carcinoid tumours, and paraneoplastic syndromes. Confusional states are particularly common in patients with advanced cancer. In about 50% of cases the cause of the confusional state cannot be determined (Bruera et al, 1990).

By far the commonest disorders are anxiety and depressive states attributable to the emotional impact of primary cancer and its recurrence. In practice, however, it is often difficult to separate the emotional impact of cancer from the side-effects of treatment. An obvious example is the woman who develops breast cancer, for whom the psychological trauma of learning that she has cancer may be compounded by mourning for the loss of the whole or part of her breast.

It is important to note that approximately two-thirds of patients with cancer do *not* develop chronic psychological disorders. It is a common clinical experience that two individuals with the same type and stage of cancer who are undergoing the same treatment will differ in their psychological responses. The following examples are typical:

> Betty, a 41-year-old married woman who worked as a computer operator, noticed a lump in her breast while taking a shower. She consulted her family doctor, who referred her to an oncology unit where a diagnosis of breast cancer was made. After the initial shock of the diagnosis, she became anxious, sad, and tearful, and found it difficult to get off to sleep. However, three weeks later, following surgery and the commencement of chemotherapy and tamoxifen, Betty's anxiety and depression subsided, and she reported (and her husband confirmed) that she was coping well and was back to her old self.

> Jane, a 43-year-old divorced woman, was a social worker. She too discovered a breast lump which turned out to be cancer. Like Betty, her cancer was at an early stage and

had not spread. Jane received exactly the same treatment as Betty. However, despite these similarities, Jane's psychological response to the diagnosis of cancer was quite different. She became increasingly anxious and preoccupied with fear that the cancer would return, and she examined her body four or five times each day to check for lumps. She was tense, restless, and unable to lead a normal life because of intrusive thoughts about cancer. She also complained of poor sleep and poor appetite. At least once a week she consulted her family doctor requesting reassurance that the cancer had not recurred. When she was first seen in Psychological Medicine, she had been in this distressed state for nearly 4 months.

Many such examples could be cited. What are the reasons for the individual differences in psychological response to cancer? This intriguing question has important clinical implications, for it leads directly to the possibility of designing effective psychological therapy. Our own work and that of others, especially the landmark studies of stress by Lazarus and Folkman (1984), indicate that a major determinant of any given patient's psychological response is the way in which the threat of cancer is perceived (appraised), together with the particular coping skills which that person can use to reduce that threat. In this book, we examine this theme in some detail and describe the ensuing development of psychological therapy specifically designed for patients with cancer.

Chapter 2

A cognitive model of adjustment to cancer

The descriptions in the previous chapter of the different reactions of Betty and Jane to the diagnosis of breast cancer illustrate well the central role that meaning plays in adjustment to serious illness. Although both women had the same good prognosis, Betty felt able to cope but Jane did not. After an initial period of confusion and distress, Betty actively engaged in her treatment, believing that she could deal with the problems that cancer posed and recover from the disease. Jane, on the other hand, was unable to get the cancer out of her mind. She was overwhelmed by thoughts about the possibility that it might recur. Cognitive models of adjustment and coping all assume that it is the interpretations we make about stressful events that determine how we respond to them (Lazarus and Folkman, 1984; Folkman and Greer, 2000). When faced with cancer some individuals, like Betty, may see the diagnosis as a challenge which they feel equipped to handle. Others, like Jane, may see it as such a huge threat that they do not have the resources to cope. Still others view the harm as already done, and perceive cancer not as a threat but as a death sentence.

Cancer threatens fundamental assumptions about our lives. Deeply held beliefs about ourselves, the world and our relationships suddenly come into question. If we have believed that we are strong, how do we manage the debilitating effects of chemotherapy? If we have strongly valued our appearance, how do we now view ourselves after a mastectomy? What happens to the sense that the world is a benevolent and just place? Some of the assumptions that are challenged by a diagnosis of cancer are universal. Some are very personal. We have found it useful to differentiate between the impact that the disease has on beliefs about survival and on beliefs about who we are.

The threat to survival

Although we may be aware that one in three of us will develop cancer at some time in our life, we usually operate as if we are somehow immune to it. People generally see themselves as less likely than others to be victims of diseases, crimes, and accidents, and have overly optimistic expectations about the future

(Perloff, 1983, 1987; Taylor and Armor, 1996). Most of us have great difficulty imagining the end of our life. As Freud wrote, it is 'impossible to imagine our own death; and whenever we attempt to do so we can perceive that we are in fact still present as spectators' (Freud, 1953). Some researchers suggest that we normally have silent assumptions that we are both invulnerable and immortal (Janoff-Bulman, 1999). We tacitly believe that the world is a just place and that we are essentially in control. These assumptions are shattered by the diagnosis of cancer. The initial reaction to this diagnosis, as Greer (1985) remarked, is to view the diagnosis of cancer as a 'catastrophic threat tantamount to a death sentence.' The initial period after the diagnosis is marked by confusion and a chaotic jumble of thoughts and feelings. There is also usually a sense of numbness, with times of great emotional turmoil alternating with a deadening of feelings ('This can't be happening to me'). From a cognitive perspective, this is the result of core beliefs about the self, the world, and the future being challenged. At first it is difficult to make sense of what is happening. Over the weeks to months following a diagnosis of cancer, patients begin to answer three vital questions about what the illness means:

1. How great is the threat?
2. What can be done about it?
3. What is the prognosis?

The threat that a diagnosis of cancer represents can be interpreted in several different ways (see Figure 2.1). It can be seen as a challenge, it can be seen as a major threat which can overwhelm or destroy, or it can be seen as harm, loss, or defeat. A fourth possibility exists, namely denial, or refusal to accept that the threat exists at all.

The personal meaning of cancer for an individual will be an important factor in determining their adjustment to the disease.

Lazarus and Folkman (1984) have contributed greatly to our understanding of how people cope with stress by demonstrating the role of appraisals in the coping process. As well as this primary appraisal of the nature of the stress,

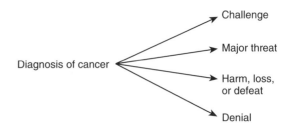

Fig. 2.1 Appraisal of the diagnosis of cancer.

a secondary appraisal takes place. This corresponds to our second question: What can be done about it? Patients vary in their beliefs about the extent to which they, or anyone else, can control or alter the disease process. Those who report the use of coping strategies as attempts to control the disease have been found to have a greater fighting spirit, are more confident of being cured, and use more active coping strategies (Link et al, 2004).

The answer to the third question (What is the prognosis?) arises from the answers to the first two questions. If the disease represents a challenge that can be met, the patient feels optimistic. If it is seen as a loss and the individual feels helpless in the face of it, the future will look very bleak. The patterns of thoughts, feelings, and behaviours associated with these appraisals represent the style of adjustment that the person develops.

Greer and Watson (1987) have identified five common adjustment styles:

1. fighting spirit
2. avoidance or denial
3. fatalism
4. helplessness and hopelessness
5. anxious preoccupation.

Fighting spirit

The person sees the illness as a challenge, and has a positive attitude towards the outcome. They engage in various behaviours, such as seeking appropriate (but not excessive) information about the disease, taking an active role in their recovery, and attempting to live as normal a life as possible.

The diagnosis is perceived as a challenge, the individual can exert some control over the stress, and the prognosis is seen as optimistic.

Typical statements made by a patient with a fighting spirit might be as follows:

'I don't dwell on my illness.'
'I try to carry on my life as I've always done.'
'I see my illness as a challenge.'
'I keep quite busy so I don't have to think about it.'

Avoidance or denial

The person denies the impact of the disease. The threat from the diagnosis is minimized, and consequently the issue of control is irrelevant and the prognosis is seen as good. The attitude of denial is accompanied by behaviour that minimizes the impact of the disease on the patient's life.

These patients make statements such as the following:

'They just took my breast off as a precaution.'
'It wasn't that serious.'

A more conscious form of this adjustment style, which has been termed *positive avoidance,* is encouraged in adjuvant psychological therapy. This involves trying to get on with life without thinking about cancer, and using distraction.

Fatalism

The patient considers that the diagnosis represents a relatively minor threat, that no control can be exerted over the situation, and that the consequences of lack of control can and should be accepted with equanimity. They have an attitude of passive acceptance. Active strategies for fighting the cancer are absent.

The person may make statements such as the following:

'It's all in the hands of the doctors/God/fate.'
'I've had a good life – what's left is a bonus.'

Helplessness and hopelessness

In this adjustment style, the patient is overwhelmed and engulfed by the enormity of the threat of cancer. Their focus of attention may be on the impending loss of life or on the illness as a defeat. The diagnosis is seen as a major threat, loss, or defeat, there is a belief that no control can be exerted over the situation, and the perceived negative outcome is experienced as if it has already occurred. Active strategies for fighting the cancer are absent, and there may be a reduction in other normal activities. The patient basically gives up.

The person who is helpless and hopeless may make statements such as the following:

'There's nothing I can do to help myself.'
'What's the point in going on?'

Anxious preoccupation

Anxiety is the predominant affect in this adjustment style. The behavioural component is one of compulsive searching for reassurance. Much of the time is spent worrying about the possibility of the disease recurring, and any physical symptoms are immediately identified as signs of new disease. Reassurance is sought by self-referral, use of alternative medicine, and excessive searching for information about cancer. The diagnosis represents a major threat, there is uncertainty about the possibility of exerting control over the situation, and the future is seen as unpredictable.

Typical statements made by the anxiously preoccupied patient include the following:

'I worry about the cancer returning or getting worse.'
'I have difficulty believing this has happened to me.'
'I can't cope with not knowing what the future holds.'

Adjustment style and psychological well-being

There is considerable evidence that an individual's attitude towards cancer is associated with their overall psychological adjustment. In early-stage cancer, an optimistic view of the future is associated with better quality of life in people with breast cancer (Carver et al, 1993), head and neck cancer (Allison et al, 2000), and prostate cancer (Roesch et al, 2005), and fighting spirit has been consistently shown to correlate with lower levels of anxiety and depression (Watson et al, 1988, 1990), Women with breast cancer who have a greater perception of control over the disease show better adjustment (Taylor et al, 1984), Finally, there is a consistent finding that active, problem-focused modes of coping are associated with better adjustment, and that the use of avoidance is associated with poorer adjustment (Heim et al, 1997; Roesch et al, 2005).

In an interesting study, female college students who scored high on a measure of hope were asked to imagine how they would cope with cancer. They were more knowledgeable about cancer and described more hope-specific coping responses than college students who were generally less hopeful (Irving et al, 1998). Cancer patients with a helpless-hopeless or anxiously preoccupied adjustment style are more likely to be depressed or anxious (Osborne et al, 1999).

The threat to the self

For some people it is not the threat of extinction which is the most frightening aspect of a diagnosis of cancer, but rather the effect that the disease has on their life. The morbidity of the disease can sometimes prove more difficult to cope with than the fear of death. Symptoms of cancer may be painful and debilitating, like those of many other diseases, and treatment may also cause suffering. Figure 2.2 shows a simple schematic representation of the very real negative consequences of the diagnosis of cancer.

Symptoms of the disease and its treatment can be aversive in a variety of different ways. They may cause pain, weakness and lethargy, nausea and vomiting, impaired concentration, and impaired mobility. These can in turn cause major disruption to the patient's lifestyle. Previously rewarding activities may

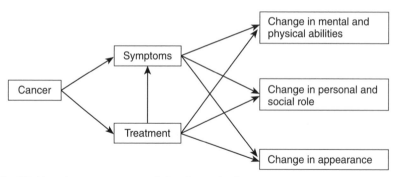

Fig. 2.2 Negative consequences of the diagnosis of cancer.

need to be reduced or even abandoned, sometimes permanently. This does not just apply to specific activities, but may also require more general changes in role. Work may no longer be possible, and for younger patients many of the demands of parenting may be too great. The results of physical disability and behavioural limitation can require adjustments of family roles on the part of both the patient and other family members. Even if the patient is relatively well, treatment sometimes has drastic effects on their bodily appearance, ranging from the temporary hair loss caused by radiotherapy and chemotherapy to permanent change after surgical treatments. Hair loss is associated with depression, loss of confidence, and shame, and for some women with breast cancer it may be more distressing than the loss of a breast. It is the most feared side-effect of chemotherapy for 56% of women, and as many as 8% may be at risk of refusing chemotherapy because of this fear (Freedman, 1994). Surgery for breast cancer can have lasting negative effects (Harcourt and Rumsey, 2001). One study found that 6 months after a mastectomy, 63% of women felt comfortable when fully dressed but only 21% felt comfortable when undressed (Harcourt et al, 2003). Moorey (2007) has published a review of the impact of breast cancer on body image.

As with the threat of death, it is the appraisal of these effects of cancer that shapes the patient's emotional reaction. Most, although by no means all, men can accept baldness as a side-effect of chemotherapy, because being bald is a socially acceptable state for men. However, women, for whom appearance is socially much more important, consider the loss of their hair a much greater threat to their self-image (Freedman, 1994). Other consequences of cancer may play into more idiosyncratic belief systems which do not fit cultural norms. For a woman to whom appearance is of central importance, the removal of a small skin tumour might cause extreme distress, even if the scarring is only minimal. For a man to whom work is the most important thing in life, a 3-month period of sickness could be catastrophic, even if he can be assured that the cancer will be cured. The threats that cancer poses to appearance, physical and mental ability, and social role will therefore affect individuals differently depending on the importance that they attach to these factors. What we have termed 'threats to the self' could also be called 'threats to the personal domain.' Beck (1976) has written extensively about the way in which 'a person's emotional response . . . depends on whether he perceives events as adding to, subtracting from, endangering or impinging upon his domain.' The personal domain refers to those aspects of his life – both tangible and intangible – which an individual perceives as having direct relevance to himself (e.g. family, friends, possessions, values, goals). Silberfarb and Greer (1982) identified four common emotional reactions to cancer, namely anxiety, anger, guilt, and depression. The particular interpretations that are made by the patient about cancer give rise to these emotions, and they can be seen as interpretations of particular threats to the personal domain.

Anxiety

The key elements of anxiety are *danger* and *vulnerability*.

These two themes are necessary to the individual's interpretation of a situation if they are to experience anxiety. Danger is present if the situation is perceived as threatening to the person's physical or social well-being, whereas vulnerability describes the perception that there are not sufficient resources to deal with the threat. When assessing risk we take account of how likely it is that the negative event will occur, as well as how bad it will be if it does occur. Even a low probability of recurrence can be intolerable if the consequences of recurrence are seen as awful and terrible. The resources available to deal with the threat will diminish anxiety. If we believe that oncologists can cure our cancer we will feel less anxious, but if we do not trust them the threat will increase. If we find it hard to have faith in our own coping abilities, this will also increase our fear.

As we have seen, death is not the only thing that people with cancer fear. The possibility of physical impairment, disfigurement, or invalidity can be a source of great anxiety. Patients who have panic attacks may believe that the bodily symptoms which they are experiencing signify impending madness. Mothers who are overprotective may become preoccupied with how their children will cope if they die, whereas overly self-reliant people may panic at the thought of the loss of control that their illness implies.

Anger

The key element here is *unjustified attack*.

Anger is generated if the person believes that their personal domain has been attacked in some way. This may be a direct attack on their physical safety or on their self-esteem, or it may be a more indirect attack on certain rules or values which the person holds dear. The angry person is primarily concerned by the unjustness of the threat that is being faced, whereas the anxious person is more concerned by the possible effects of the threat on their personal safety. A focus on future pain and inability to cope creates anxiety. If the patient thinks about the doctor's failure to control the pain or about life's unfairness in making them suffer, they are more likely to become angry. This sense that an agent (personal or impersonal) is abusing them seems to be one of the basic requirements for an angry reaction. People may become angry with God for his failure to save them, or with their partner for not providing adequate support. Having the illness may lead them to identify with other people's suffering, allowing them to become angry about health service cuts or a child's death as if these affected them directly.

By focusing on external violations of their rights, the angry person is thinking less about personal vulnerability or imperfection. It is possible to become locked in an angry mode, and for this to provide a form of defence against some of the more unpleasant consequences of the disease itself. A woman who had hormone-dependent breast cancer made repeated complaints about not receiving treatments to which she felt that she was entitled. These included hormonal treatments and counselling. It is likely that she was working on a rule such as 'I am entitled to the best treatment available, and if I do not get it this is because it is being deliberately withheld.' Her hostile strategy had the effect of both mobilizing her energy to fight the disease, and preventing her from focusing too closely on its effects.

The decision as to whether or not a belief is maladaptive is not an easy one, and cannot be made simply on the basis that the belief is irrational. In this woman's case, her anger could be seen as having both adaptive and maladaptive functions. In fact, some studies have provided evidence that these 'hostile patients', who are often labelled as 'difficult' by their doctors, survive longer than more compliant patients (Derogatis et al, 1979). On the other hand, a study by Taylor et al (1984) indicated that women with breast cancer who blamed others had poorer psychological adjustment. Sadness and fear are socially acceptable emotions to relatives of patients, but anger presents more problems.

Guilt

The key element here is *self-blame.*

The guilty person, like the angry one, is concerned with apportioning blame. An important rule has been violated, and someone is responsible. The difference is that the guilty person blames him- or herself. Guilt often exists as part of a depressive picture. However, it may occur independently, and when this happens it is often a result of the person's attempt to give meaning to their experience. In the search for an explanation for the illness, people with cancer may decide that they have brought it on themselves and that they are being punished for some sin or crime. If they can find some way of expiating their sin, or of gaining control over the disease, they may be able to overcome the guilt. However, if they are unable to do this, they may become fixated on the past and ruminate about the way they have ruined their life ('If only I hadn't done that, I might not have become ill'). Thoughts such as 'I'm a burden' or 'I've brought this on my family' result in guilt and self-reproach about the effect of cancer on others. If the person with cancer has a rule that they are responsible for what people close to them feel, or that it is their job to prevent their family from feeling unhappy, they may feel guilty about having cancer. Rather than blaming the disease for the family's suffering, the person with cancer may unfairly blame him- or herself.

Sadness and depression

The key element here is *loss or defeat*.

The theme of sadness is loss from the personal domain. The losses in cancer are self-evident – loss of parts of the body, loss of strength and vitality, and loss of valued role. The real losses which occur as a result of the objective consequences of the disease only cause a depressed mood if they are perceived as important by the patient. Loss of hair is not significant to someone who attaches little value to physical appearance, and the opportunity to give up work may be welcomed by some people. It is only if the loss impinges on the personal domain that it produces sadness. If these reactions become enduring ways of viewing the self, they become integrated into the person's self-concept.

Information processing in cancer

Once a negative view of the disease and its impact on the individual has established itself, it tends to be self-perpetuating. Normally we have a slight selective bias for positive information. Taylor and Armor (1996) suggest that when a person faces negative or threatening events, these positive assessments of self, personal control, and optimism about the future are challenged. An attempt is made to restore or enhance the positive perceptions, leading to 'positive illusions' in the face of adversity. For instance, patients with heart disease and AIDS tend to compare themselves with patients they view as less fortunate than themselves (Helgeson and Taylor, 1993; Taylor et al, 1993). People with a fighting spirit may be more optimistic about their prognosis than is appropriate in the circumstances, although this can often be perceived as choosing to see the glass as half full rather than half empty, rather than an *illusory* view of their situation. This tendency to put the most positive spin on the implications of cancer for self-perception, self-control, and view of the future is usually associated with better adjustment and a more active coping style (Taylor and Armor, 1996). Whereas a confirmatory positive bias may be present in people who show good psychological adaptation, there certainly seems to be a negative bias in those who exhibit maladaptive adjustment styles. Their negative schemata process information in such a way as to maintain their negative view of themselves or their survival. People with cancer who become depressed or anxious distort information in a similar way to other depressed or anxious patients. Numerous studies have demonstrated this cognitive bias (for a literature review, see Clark and Steer, 1996). The process of distorting this information in a negative way often involves systematic logical errors or cognitive distortions, the commonest of which have been identified by Beck et al (1979), and are described below.

All-or-nothing thinking

In this type of cognitive distortion, events are seen as black and white, with no shades of grey. For instance, a person may conclude that because his cancer cannot be cured, he might as well give up and die. The disease is perceived as either cure or death, whereas the reality might be months or years of remission. An athletic person might conclude 'If I'm not well enough to play football, I can get no pleasure from anything.'

Selective abstraction

Here the person selects part of the information available to suit their predominant cognitive set. When having a treatment explained to them, an anxious person may hear that it is painful and unpleasant, but will pay less attention to the fact that it has a high chance of being successful. The depressed person with breast cancer focuses on the loss of her breast, but pays little attention to the fact that her husband still finds her sexually attractive.

Arbitrary inference

The uncertainty that surrounds the cancer prognosis means that there is often insufficient evidence on which to base judgements about the future. Patients may still come to arbitrary conclusions that the disease will inevitably recur and kill them. As well as jumping to conclusions, patients make arbitrary inferences about other people's thoughts and motivations (mind reading). Harmless looks are interpreted as indicating that the relative knows something bad but will not disclose it.

Overgeneralization

In this type of cognitive distortion, a single negative event is seen as a never-ending pattern. For instance, on her return from hospital a woman with ovarian cancer has her first argument with her husband. She thinks to herself 'We'll never stop arguing – our marriage is over.'

Labelling

Labelling ignores the fact that people are complex mixtures of characteristics. Instead, it defines them in terms of a single global construct. Statements such as 'I'm just a chronic invalid' or 'Nurses are angels' indicate that labelling is taking place.

Magnification and minimization

In this type of cognitive distortion, certain pieces of the perceptual field are enlarged or reduced in perspective in order to suit the person's cognitive set. In depression, for instance, the chances of a remission from the cancer might be minimized in the person's mind. Someone who is denying her problems will minimize the seriousness of the symptoms ('They only took my breast off as a precaution'), whereas an anxious person might magnify the pain of an injection.

These thinking errors cause the person with cancer to misinterpret or bias their judgements about the disease. In people with a maladaptive adjustment style, these processing biases produce *negative automatic thoughts*. These are idiosyncratic, plausible thoughts which come into consciousness unbidden. They contain logical errors in their reasoning, but to the person who is experiencing them they seem accurate and realistic. It is often only when the individual is removed from the stressful situation that these thoughts can be seen to be irrational.

Typical automatic thoughts include the following:

'I can never be happy again.'
'It's no good fighting – you always get knocked for six.'
'I can't cope.'
'I hate myself.'
'The doctors only want to use me as a guinea pig.'
'I'm not a real man/woman any more.'

An automatic thought is a thought or image that is not necessarily at the centre of the person's attention, but which is accessible to consciousness. These thoughts, together with the emotions and behaviours with which they are associated, are the key components of cognitive behavioural therapy (CBT). Psychodynamic therapies make interpretations and inferences about unconscious processes. Cognitive therapies make use of conscious cognitions. Dreams may be the royal road to the unconscious, but thoughts give entry to the rules and meaning systems that govern our feelings and actions.

Thoughts, feelings, behaviour, and physiology

The discussion so far has given cognition a central place in adjustment to cancer. The view that a person takes of the meaning of cancer directly influences their emotional and behavioural reactions, particularly their attempts at coping, but the relationship is not simply one-directional. There is a complex interplay between thoughts, feelings, behaviour, and physical reactions, in which no single component has primacy (see Figure 2.3). For instance, thoughts such as 'What's the point? I'm never going to get through this, it's hopeless', will not only increase a person's feelings of depression, but will also decrease their motivation, so that they give up their social activities. With less opportunity to meet friends and relatives there is more time for negative thinking, less pleasure, and so the hopeless thoughts are confirmed and the mood becomes even lower. Depressed mood is often associated with fatigue and lethargy.

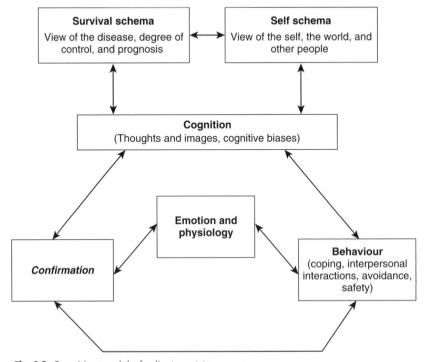

Fig. 2.3 Cognitive model of adjustment to cancer.

These physical symptoms can be misinterpreted as evidence that the disease is worsening, reinforcing hopelessness and depression. Chapter 4 considers how mental processes may have a direct effect on the progression of cancer.

The role of family and friends

The interaction of the person with cancer with other people influences both the impact of the effects of the disease and the person's ability to cope with them. Family relationships can be dramatically changed as a result of the disease. The affected partner may have to give up the role of caregiver, bread-winner, or supporter in the family. This may have wider implications for the quality of the family relationship.

The effects of the real changes brought about by the illness will again be determined by the personal meanings that they hold for all of the actors in the drama. This involves the meaning of pain, debility, and role change not only for the person with cancer, but also for other family members. Thus a complex interaction between the disease and members of the family, as well as between the family members themselves, is set up.

Much interest has been generated by the idea that social support can buffer the patient against some of the stresses of cancer. Some workers have predicted that patients with a wider social network or one that provides higher levels of emotional support will be better adjusted to the disease, and there does seem to be some evidence for this (Helgeson and Cohen, 1996). It is often the extent and quality of *perceived* support, rather than the objective level of support, that is most important (Bloom, 1986). In breast cancer, social support is associated with more positive reframing and less self-blame (Kim et al, 2010), while women who experience more emotional/instrumental support are more hope-ful. Psychological distress is related to decreased emotional support by the partner over time (Brady and Hegeson, 1999), and women with a high depres-sion burden have been found to consistently lose more network members than women who experienced depression but did not rank it among the top five side-effects of cancer (Badger et al, 1999).

The ability of family members to provide emotional support depends upon their own reaction to the disease. On the one hand, a husband who is so fright-ened by the thought of cancer that he believes nothing can be done to help will be ineffectual in helping his wife to fight the disease. On the other hand, a hus-band who believes that patients must be cared for and should not be expected to do anything would also limit his wife's ability to function well. Renneker (1982) describes a husband who believed so strongly that cancer was incurable that he went out of his way to prevent his wife receiving treatment that might have been curative.

Again it might be predicted that it is the partner's thoughts about cancer and the patient's role in the family that determine their emotional response. Coursey et al (1975) found that anxiety is often greater in immediate family members than in patients themselves. The partner goes through the same reactions to cancer as the patient, but their need to provide support often prevents them from being able to express their feelings openly. During treatment the patient may no longer be able to carry out their normal role, and the stresses on the partner may consequently be great. Sometimes this results in observable depression or anxiety in the partner, but more commonly it is manifested as problems in the relationship. For example, a patient with lung metastases from breast cancer had always been the dominant partner. Her increasing breathlessness and disability threw her husband into a panic. He compensated by becoming the perfect nurse, constantly at her bedside, attending to her every need. However, periodically his own need for dependence would emerge and he would collapse. This resulted in his wife resuming her dominant role briefly, until the cycle repeated itself. This unsatisfactory state of affairs continued until her death.

Another way in which partners cope with stress is by clinging to patterns of behaviour that were used before the cancer was diagnosed, refusing to alter their habits and pretending that nothing has changed. The husband of a woman with breast cancer habitually reacted to stress and conflict by avoiding and ignoring them. He refused to visit his wife in hospital. When she came home he made no allowances for her illness, expecting her to look after the house and the children as before. Although she was not seriously physically ill, she felt tired and frightened. His inability to face the illness meant that she had no one to help her to cope with her emotional burden. In addition, he expected her to carry on with no change in her daily routine, despite her fatigue.

Another type of problem arises when the illness upsets the balance of power or sharing of responsibility within the relationship. Resentment can occur on both sides as a result of this upset.

The effect of cancer on sexual function has already been described. People with cancer often perceive themselves as less sexually attractive or, more subtly, see themselves as less potent or less feminine. These problems are compounded if communication difficulties ensue. A common example of this is the husband who does not initiate lovemaking after his wife's mastectomy because he is not sure that she is well enough. If he does not give his reasons, the wife may misinterpret his behaviour as a sign that he no longer finds her sexually attractive. When he does show an interest in sex she rebuffs him, hurting his feelings and reducing the likelihood that he will initiate further lovemaking.

Changes in the disease may exacerbate existing marital difficulties. These too can be understood in cognitive terms. Couples often operate on the basis of unrealistic rules or beliefs about each other. For instance, a person might believe that 'My partner should know what is important to me without my having to tell him or her.' The onset of illness throws this system into stark relief, since there are now many new feelings and symptoms which the partner is expected to immediately know about and be able to read in the patient. People close to the patient, particularly their partner and family, but also doctors and nurses, have a significant effect on their emotional state. Interaction with strangers and acquaintances can be nearly as important in some cases. For example, in a study that assessed the thoughts evoked by being in a situation with a disabled person whom one does not know well, Fichten (1986) found that anxiety was high, negative thoughts about the other person were prominent, and self-efficacy beliefs were low compared with an interaction with an able-bodied person. Similar processes probably occur when healthy people meet others with cancer, particularly those with an obvious health disability. Feelings of embarrassment and discomfort can lead to reduced contact with an acquaintance who has cancer, resulting in increasing social isolation.

It is remarkable how well many relatives cope with the burdens that cancer places on them. In some cases, marriages may actually improve as a result of one partner having cancer (Hughes, 1987), and despite the enormous strains involved, the divorce rates for long-term survivors do not appear to be higher than those for the normal population (Fobair et al, 1986). The cognitive model must therefore take account of interpersonal factors that influence the individual's reaction. Interactions with family, friends, professionals, and strangers can all be significant. A series of interactions occur between the person and others which affect that person's perceptions of the real consequences of the disease, as well as his or her ability to cope. This is a flexible and fluid process. A change in any part of the system, whether it is a deterioration in physical health or a difference in the level of support received, inevitably has effects on the other components. It is the way in which these changes are actively cognitively processed that determines the final psychological reaction. In Chapter 11 we shall demonstrate how this theoretical framework has been used to construct a psychological treatment for couples who are facing the stresses of cancer.

Vulnerability to adjustment disorders

Although CBT is primarily focused on the individual's reaction to the threats posed by cancer in the present, it does not ignore the influence of *past* experience on current appraisal and coping processes. Our fundamental beliefs about the world are formed from childhood experiences. If our parenting was good, we will usually develop a sense that others are helpful and supportive, that the world is a relatively benign place where we can exert some control, and that we are worthwhile. As Janoff-Bulman (1999) has pointed out, these beliefs are irrevocably changed by traumatic experience. Most people are able to adapt their world view in the light of this new experience so that they see the world as both benign *and* potentially dangerous. Even some time after traumatic events, survivors' assumptions are less positive than those of the general population (Janoff-Bulman, 1992). The more rigid and absolute these beliefs about a just and controllable world are, the more difficult it will be to incorporate traumatic events into the world view, or schema. This may lead to a sudden shift to a set of beliefs that the world is unjust and uncontrollable, and the development of the maladaptive adjustment styles described earlier in this chapter.

Cognitive psychologists, building on the work of Bartlett (1932), have used the concept of a *schema* as a means of understanding how mental processes make sense of the world and make plans for action. A schema can be defined as 'a relatively enduring structure that functions like a template; it actively screens, codes, categorizes, and evaluates information. By definition it also represents some relevant prior experiences' (Kovacs and Beck, 1978, p. 00). The threat of cancer challenges schemas relating to a person's very existence and basic beliefs about him- or herself, and the person is forced to modify or develop a new set of beliefs.

Not all core beliefs are positive initially. Alongside experiences of being loved and valued, most of us have experienced negative events in our lives that have led us to doubt our worth, our competence, and our trust in others. If the experience of having cancer confirms these hidden doubts, a dormant negative schema may be activated. For instance, if a man witnessed constant arguments and violence between his parents when he was a child, he might develop a basic belief that the world is a chaotic and unpredictable place where bad things happen. However, over the course of his life he may develop a coping strategy of establishing control, elaborating a secondary belief that if he can control his life, he will be safe. The unpredictability of cancer threatens this fragile coping strategy, and his core beliefs about the world will resurface, leading to the development of helplessness/hopelessness or anxious preoccupation. Other cognitive therapists have developed similar models linking past experiences, underlying beliefs, and people's reactions to illness (Williams, 1997; White, 2001).

The clinical relevance of the cognitive model will be expanded throughout Part Two of this book. The next two chapters will review the research relating to adjustment styles and the effectiveness of psychological therapy for cancer patients.

Summary

1. Cancer is a disease that poses a severe threat to many aspects of the individual's life.

2. It is not the objective consequences of the disease as such but rather the way in which they are interpreted which determines the individual's reactions.

3. Emotional reactions are determined by the particular threat that cancer represents to the individual's personal domain. Core positive beliefs about the self, the world, and others are challenged, and core negative beliefs are activated.

4. The content of emotional reactions can be understood in terms of the cognitive processes that are taking place.

5. The individual's adjustment to the disease is a result of the interaction between the interpretation of the stresses involved and the coping strategies that are available.

6. The individual's adjustment to the disease is influenced by the quality of the emotional support that is available.

Chapter 3

Can CBT improve quality of life?

There is now a considerable body of evidence concerning the effectiveness of psychological therapy in people with cancer. This ranges from clinical case reports and single case studies to large well-designed randomized controlled trials. Evaluating this evidence poses some problems, because the studies have not all asked the same research questions, and the target patient populations often differ in various respects, so direct comparisons are not always possible. In fact, the question 'Can CBT improve quality of life?' proves to be too general. Most trials have looked at anxiety, depression, and adjustment to the disease as indicators of quality of life, but other factors such as interpersonal and social functioning have been less closely investigated, and more recently investigators have begun to focus on packages for specific symptoms such as insomnia and fatigue. A psychological therapy could have more of an effect on some of these factors than on others. Aspects of the disease and the patient group could also influence the effectiveness of therapy. Many studies have used a mixed sample of cancer patients. This design can obscure differential effects of treatment on different diagnostic groups, and it is only possible to perform an analysis of subgroups if the sample is large. For instance, Edgar et al (1992) found that the superiority of an early intervention over a late one, which applied to the whole sample, did not apply to patients with breast cancer. However, when a single diagnostic group is investigated, it may be difficult to generalize the findings to other groups. A second important variable is the level of psychological distress. Most studies have taken all patients without selecting for psychological morbidity. However, there does seem to be evidence that psychological therapy is of more benefit to people who are in a state of distress (Sheard and Maguire, 1999). Indeed, a study of group psychotherapy in patients with primary non-metastatic breast cancer reported that therapy had no significant effect in well-adjusted (i.e. non-distressed) patients (Vos et al, 2007).

Side-effects of treatment and stage of disease could also influence the effects of psychological therapy. Therapy might well be helpful for people with early-stage disease and a good prognosis, but not for those with terminal illness. Because studies have taken various cancer diagnoses and intervened at different stages of the disease, they cannot be easily compared, and conclusions at the moment are tentative. With the exception of certain research groups that have carried out a systematic programme of investigation (e.g. Fawzy and colleagues, Cunningham and colleagues, and Greer and colleagues), most reports are of one-off trials, so our knowledge of the area is being built up in a relatively piecemeal fashion.

Because our intervention is a cognitive behavioural treatment, we shall focus mainly on the evidence for the effectiveness of CBT. Only randomized controlled trials of treatment have been included in this review.

Individual CBT

Weisman and Worden (Weisman et al, 1980) were among the first to systematically conduct research on psychological treatment in people with cancer. They initially devised a psychological screening instrument that predicted emotional distress (Weisman and Worden, 1977), and then assessed patients with newly diagnosed cancers of the breast, colon, lung, or female reproductive tract, or with newly diagnosed Hodgkin's disease and malignant melanoma. One-third of the patients ($n = 125$) were found to be at high risk of emotional distress, but only 59 patients were eventually given psychological treatment, since 28 individuals refused to participate and 38 individuals were excluded on other grounds.

The patients were then randomly allocated to four sessions of consultation therapy or cognitive skills training. Consultation therapy consisted of helping patients to identify problems, encouraging the ventilation of feelings associated with these problems, and exploring ways of solving the problems, preferably by direct confrontation. Emphasis was placed on the patient's personal control and competence. This patient-centred individualized approach was compared with cognitive skills training, which focused on the general process of psychosocial problem solving. The therapist first taught a step-by-step approach to problem solving by means of paired cards that depicted cancer-related problems and how these could be solved. Patients practised this approach and learned how to apply it to their own specific problems. Cognitive skills training also included relaxation training. Patients received homework assignments related to relaxation and problem solving. Both of these therapies contained elements which can be found in adjuvant psychological therapy (APT). Cognitive skills training contained structure and specific CBT techniques, and consultation therapy contained problem solving, emotional expression, and enhancement of personal control.

Patients in the treatment group were compared with an untreated control group of patients from an earlier study who were at high risk of emotional distress. When the patients were assessed 2 to 6 months after diagnosis, the two psychological treatments were found to be equally effective in relieving emotional distress and improving psychosocial problem solving. This trial was a groundbreaking example of psychosocial research in oncology, in its development of a screening instrument for emotional distress, its detailed description of therapy, its random allocation to treatment, and its use of an untreated control group. However, there were two methodological shortcomings.

1. The untreated control group was obtained from an earlier study, and was therefore not randomly allocated.

2. Of the total study sample ($n = 125$), less than 50% ($n = 59$) actually took part in the treatment trial.

Linn et al (1982) investigated the impact of counselling on adjustment in men with cancer who were judged to have a life expectancy of 3–12 months. Patients were randomly assigned to either a treatment group or an untreated control group. Although not designated as CBT, counselling included a mixture of non-directive and cognitive behavioural strategies similar to those used in APT. Therapists set out to reduce denial but to maintain hope, encourage meaningful activities, reinforce accomplishments, and increase self-esteem. In keeping with the late and often terminal stage of cancer treated in this study, the therapy often involved *being with* as much as *doing to* the patient: 'simply listening, understanding, and sometimes only sitting quietly with the patient were elements of treatment … the therapist was often with the patient at the time of death.' Three months after the start of counselling the treated patients were less depressed, had higher self-esteem, and had an increased internal locus of control in comparison with the untreated controls.

Using an interesting study design, Edgar et al (1992) compared CBT delivered early with CBT delivered later in the first year after diagnosis. A total of 205 patients with various cancers were contacted as soon after diagnosis as possible, and were randomly allocated to either an early intervention group which received treatment immediately, or a late intervention group which received treatment 4 months later. The early intervention group began therapy on average 11 weeks after diagnosis, and the late group commenced therapy 28 weeks after diagnosis. The intervention consisted of five sessions, each lasting for 1 hour, with a nurse. The techniques that were used included problem solving, goal setting, cognitive reappraisal, and relaxation training. A multidisciplinary workshop on the effective use of resources was also offered to patients at 4-month intervals.

Four months after diagnosis (when the early intervention group had received treatment but the late intervention group had not) there were no differences between the conditions. Eight months after diagnosis the late intervention group was significantly less depressed, anxious, and worried. At the 12-month assessment the late intervention group had less worry related to illness, but there were no other differences between the treatments. Unfortunately, this trial did not include a treatment-as-usual group, so we do not have a picture of the natural course of adjustment in this sample, and therefore cannot know whether the two methods of treatment delivery had any long-term advantage over no treatment. From these results it would appear that giving CBT later rather than sooner in the first year after diagnosis reduces distress more rapidly (although an analysis of subgroups showed that breast cancer patients did equally well in both conditions). The authors speculated that the emotional work that needs to be accomplished after diagnosis is too overwhelming to allow patients to benefit from coping skills training during the first few months. They suggest that if this approach is offered in the first few months, it may need to be continued longer until the patient can use the coping strategies. An alternative might be to incorporate more emotion-based work into the traditional CBT framework, as we have done in APT (see Chapter 7).

Elsesser et al (1994) conducted a small study that compared a combination of anxiety management and stress inoculation training with a waiting-list control in people with various cancer diagnoses. There were slight improvements on psychological variables in the treatment group.

Randomized controlled trials of adjuvant psychological therapy

The first evaluation of our own treatment was a prospective randomized controlled trial comparing APT with treatment as usual (Greer et al, 1992). Patients aged between 18 and 74 years who were attending the Royal Marsden Hospital at the time of diagnosis or first recurrence of cancer were screened for psychological morbidity. To ensure that there was a large enough sample for follow-up, only people with a life expectancy of at least 12 months were eligible to participate. The participants completed the Hospital Anxiety and Depression Scale (HADS) and the Mental Adjustment to Cancer Scale (MACS). Those who scored 10 or higher on the Anxiety Scale of the HADS, or scored 8 or higher on the Depression Scale of the HADS, or scored high on helplessness/ hopelessness and low on fighting spirit on the MACS, were invited to take part in the study. Those who agreed to participate were randomly allocated to either six sessions of APT or an untreated control group. The participants in the control group were able to access the usual support of the hospital, but did not receive the structured intervention. The main outcome measures were the HADS, the MACS, the Rotterdam Symptom Checklist (RSCL), and the

Psychosocial Adjustment to Illness Scale (PAIS). Assessments were made before therapy, at 8 weeks, and at 4 months of follow-up. In total, 174 patients entered the trial, of whom 156 patients (90%) completed the 8-week trial. Follow-up data at 4 months were obtained for 137 patients (79%). At 8 weeks, patients receiving therapy had significantly higher scores than control patients on fighting spirit, and significantly lower scores on helplessness, anxious preoccupation and fatalism, anxiety, psychological symptoms, and orientation towards healthcare. At 4 months, patients receiving therapy had significantly lower scores than controls on anxiety, psychological symptoms, and psychological distress. Clinically, the proportion of severely anxious patients decreased from 46% at baseline to 20% at 8 weeks and 20% at 4 months in the therapy group, and from 48% at baseline to 41% at 8 weeks and 43% at 4 months among the controls. The proportion of patients with depression was 40% at baseline, 13% at 8 weeks, and 18% at 4 months in the therapy group, and 30% at baseline, 29% at 8 weeks, and 23% at 4 months in the controls. At 1 year there was a significant difference in change from baseline on the PAIS, and a tendency for the therapy group to show more change on measures of helplessness and anxiety (Moorey et al, 1994). Only 19% of the therapy patients were in the clinical range for anxiety, compared with 44% of the controls (see Figures 3.1 and 3.2).

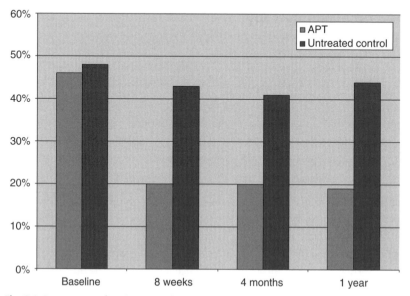

Fig. 3.1 Percentage of patients scoring > 10 on the HADS Anxiety Scale in the therapy and control groups.

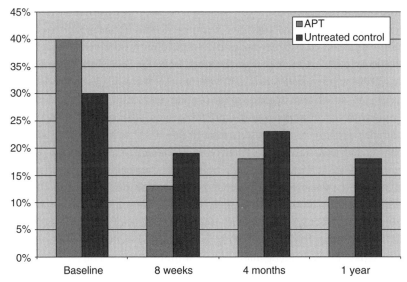

Fig. 3.2 Percentage of patients scoring > 8 on the HADS Depression Scale in the therapy and control groups.

A striking feature of this study was the high refusal rate. When the reasons for this were examined, it emerged that patients with stage I disease were most likely to refuse to participate. Patients were less likely to participate if they had low-volume disease, were receiving no further treatment, or had fewer physical symptoms. Men who scored high for anxious preoccupation were more likely to agree to take part in the study.

Having demonstrated that APT was more effective than a treatment-as-usual control, the next step was to compare the therapy with a control treatment in a clinical setting (Moorey et al, 1998). Patients were selected from the Psychological Medicine Clinic at the Royal Marsden Hospital. Patients with various cancers who had been referred for psychiatric assessment, and who met the criteria for an abnormal adjustment reaction, were randomly allocated to either 8 weeks of APT or 8 weeks of a comparison treatment consisting of supportive counselling. Both treatments were administered by ourselves. The supportive counselling (which like APT was conducted as individual weekly sessions, including the patient's partner where appropriate) was designed to control for therapist's time and attention and for non-specific factors, but to exclude techniques thought to be key ingredients of APT. Non-directive techniques were used to encourage ventilation of feelings in an empathic therapeutic relationship. Information about cancer and the nature of emotional reactions to cancer was given to the patient if they requested it, or if the need arose during the session. The counselling sessions were unstructured, with no agenda. Behavioural and cognitive techniques were not used, and no homework was assigned between sessions. Because both therapists had a strong allegiance to CBT, and neither were trained Rogerian therapists, this cannot be regarded as a full comparison of APT with another therapy. However, we believe that this approach approximates to the routine counselling that many distressed people with cancer might receive from nurses and other professionals.

Similar outcome measures were used to those in the first study. In addition to the HADS and the MACS, patients completed a measure of the types of coping strategies that are taught in APT, namely the Cancer Coping Questionnaire (CCQ). Some other measures which are more commonly used in CBT for anxiety and for depression, namely the Spielberger State-Trait Anxiety Inventory (STAI) (Spielberger et al, 1970) and the Beck Depression Inventory (BDI) (Beck et al, 1961), respectively, were included so that comparisons with other CBT studies could be made.

At 8 weeks after the baseline assessment, APT had produced a significantly greater change than the counselling intervention on fighting spirit, helplessness, coping with cancer, anxiety, and self-defined problems. At 4 months after the baseline assessment, APT had produced a significantly greater change than the counselling intervention on fighting spirit, coping with cancer, anxiety, and self-defined problems. Unfortunately, insufficient numbers of patients were available at follow-up (due to ill health or patients having moved away). These results are encouraging, as they show that APT does not simply exert its effect through non-specific factors. The change in CCQ scores in CBT but not in counselling confirms that patients do learn to think in cognitive terms and to use strategies from the therapy.

Moynihan et al (1998) evaluated APT in men with testicular cancer. Whereas the first trial had included patients with any cancer who were psychologically distressed, this trial focused on a single diagnostic group and assessed whether or not APT could help all patients, whether or not they were distressed. Patients attending the Testicular Tumour Unit at the Royal Marsden Hospital were randomly allocated to six sessions of APT or a treatment-as-usual control. In total, 73 (40%) of 184 eligible patients agreed to take part, and 81 patients (44%) did not wish to participate, but agreed to complete further assessments. A total of 30 patients wanted no further contact with the assessors. Only results for the HADS were reported. At 2 months, change from baseline favoured the treated group on the anxiety subscale, but this was not sustained when adjusted for factors related to the disease. By 12 months, change from baseline appeared to favour the control condition. The authors concluded that men with testicular cancer appear to have considerable coping abilities, and that routine psychological support was not indicated. Table 3.1 summarizes the findings from trials of individual CBT in people with cancer.

Psychoeducational groups

Heinrich and Schag (1985) compared a psychoeducational programme for patients and their partners with currently available care. A total of 494 patients were screened, of whom 92 patients fulfilled the screening criteria (Karnofsky score > 70, age 25–70 years, no major cognitive deficits, no major psychiatric illnesses, and living within 50 miles of the hospital). Of these individuals, 81 patients were contacted, and 70 patients finally entered the study. Only 51 patients completed the pre- and post-intervention evaluations. Most of the patients had been living with cancer for over 2 years. Therapy consisted of a structured small group programme. The goal of the group was to educate patients and their partners about cancer and its impact, and to teach them coping skills. The groups included education and information about cancer, relaxation training, modifications of the cognitive therapy described by Weisman et al (1980), and problem solving and activity management. Activity management included a walking exercise component and contracting for the patient and their partner to increase positively valued individual and couple activities.

Both groups improved over the course of the study, and there were no significant differences on measures of adjustment. Patients and their partners showed improvement on scores on the Cancer Information Test, indicating that the educational component of the treatment had been successful. At the post-intervention evaluation and 2-month follow-up there was a positive effect on coping in medical situations and achieving goals in the treated group. Both patients and partners reported that the education about cancer and the relaxation training were the most helpful components of the therapy. Although this intervention was targeted at partners as well as patients, only 12 partners in the treatment group and 13 partners in the control group completed the study (out of a possible 51 partners).

Telch and Telch (1986) randomized 41 outpatients with a variety of cancer types and stages to one of three groups, namely coping skills instruction, supportive therapy, and untreated control. The coping skills condition consisted of six sessions, each lasting for 90 minutes. One of the following five different instructional modes was presented each week:

1. relaxation and stress management
2. communication and assertion
3. problem solving and constructive thinking

Table 3.1 Randomized controlled trials of individual CBT in people with cancer

Study	Interventions	n	Cancer type	Stage of disease	Selection	Outcome	Follow-up
Linn et al (1982)	Counselling vs. no treatment	120	Men with various cancers	Advanced Life expectancy 3–12 months	All patients	CBT > NTC	None
Weissman et al (1980)	4 sessions comparing two CBT interventions: CST vs. CT	59	Various cancers	Newly diagnosed	Patients at high risk of emotional distress	2–6 months after diagnosis: CST = CT	None
Edgar et al (1992)	5 sessions of coping skills training administered early (EI) or late (LI)	205	Various cancers	Newly diagnosed	All patients	4 months: EI = LI	8 months: LI > EI 1 year: LI > EI
Greer et al (1992) Moorey et al (1994)	6 sessions of APT vs. treatment as usual	168	Various cancers	Newly diagnosed and recurrence	Screened patients with high levels of anxiety or depression	CBT > NTC	1 year: CBT > NTC
Elsesser (1994)	6 sessions of anxiety management training and stress inoculation training	27	Various cancers	All stages	All patients	CBT > NTC Effect only small	None

Study	Intervention	N	Cancer	Disease stage	Patient selection	Result	Follow-up
Fawzy et al (1996)	6 sessions of group CBT vs. individual CBT vs. assessment only	104	Malignant melanoma	Newly diagnosed	All patients	(group CBT = individual CBT) > NTC	1 year: group CBT > (individual CBT = NTC) Coping skills and confusion
Moynihan et al (1998)	6 sessions of APT	73	Testicular cancer	Newly diagnosed	All patients	CBT = NTC	1 year: control > CBT
Moorey et al (1998)	8 sessions of APT vs. supportive counselling	47	Various cancers	All stages of disease	Patients referred to psycho-oncology service	CBT > ST	2 months: CBT > ST
Doorenbos et al (2005)	10 sessions over 18 weeks (5 face-to-face and 5 telephone sessions) vs. treatment as usual	237	Various cancers	Early stage undergoing chemotherapy	Patients attending oncology centre	CBT > NTC for symptom limitations	None

APT, adjuvant psychological therapy; ST, supportive therapy; NTC, no-treatment control; CST, cognitive skills training; CT, consultation therapy; EI, early intervention; LI, late intervention.

4. feelings management
5. pleasant activity planning.

The participants rehearsed skills in the session through the use of structured exercises, and then practised them as homework assignments. In contrast, the support group was unstructured. The group leader acted as a facilitator, encouraging the discussion of feelings and identifying underlying themes such as helplessness and loss of control.

Patients who received supportive therapy showed little improvement, while in the untreated group there was actually a deterioration in psychological adjustment. The coping skills group showed significantly greater improvement than the other two conditions. These gains were in areas such as affect, satisfaction with work, social activities, physical appearance and sexual intimacy, communication, and coping with medical procedures. Patients kept a diary of their homework practice, and the records confirmed that most of them used the coping skills on a daily basis. The authors suggested that the support group may have been less effective because the patients were too heterogeneous and the intervention was too brief for group cohesion to have developed. Although this was an excellent study in many respects, the lack of any follow-up beyond the end of therapy assessment is a serious flaw, as there could have been a delayed effect on patients' functioning (as was found by Fawzy and Fawzy, 1994).

Over a period of two decades, Cunningham and colleagues have been developing and systematically evaluating a psychoeducational group approach to coping with cancer. Their brief intervention consists of six weekly sessions, each lasting for 2 hours. The first hour of each session is didactic (learning a specific coping skill, relaxation, use of mental imagery, cognitive restructuring, goal definition, and problem solving), while the second hour is supportive (sharing of experiences and feelings). Participants are given a workbook and two tapes, and are encouraged to practise the skills learned in the sessions as homework.

In their first controlled trial (Cunningham and Tocco, 1989) using this approach, this mixture of support and psychoeducational therapy was compared with 6 weeks of support alone. The patients consisted of 60 consecutive referrals to the coping skills training programme. The sample was heterogeneous (various diagnoses, 50% with recurrent disease and 50% currently undergoing cancer treatment). Assessments were conducted at the start and end of therapy, and again 2–3 weeks after the end of therapy. In total, 53 patients completed the trial. Both groups showed significant improvements in psychological adjustment, but the effect was greater in the psychoeducational group.

A separate group of 39 patients received the coping skills training and were not randomized; the improvements in mood were largely maintained at a 3-month follow-up. These changes appear to be mediated by changes in perceived self-efficacy (Cunningham et al, 1991), are applicable to various types of cancer and stages of disease, and can be delivered by therapists with different backgrounds (Cunningham et al, 1993).

Because it often proves difficult for patients to attend six weekly sessions because of the distance from the treatment centre or the side-effects of treatment, the research team devised an intensive weekend version of the group. Both interventions produced statistically significant improvements which persisted at a 3-month follow-up, even though the health of many of the participants deteriorated (Cunningham et al, 1995). Following the promising results of the study by Spiegel et al (1989) (see Chapter 4), which demonstrated an effect of long-term group therapy on survival of women with metastatic breast cancer, Cunningham and colleagues evaluated the effects of lengthening their programme (Edmonds et al, 1999). The longer-term group intervention consisted of 35 weekly 2-hour support groups, with a 20-week course of CBT assignments completed by patients at home and discussed in the group, and a weekend intensive coping skills course. From 130 patients who attended an intake interview, 66 patients were finally randomized into the study. In total, 30 patients received the intervention and 36 patients were in the control group. The control subjects received treatment as usual as well as the workbook and audiotapes that were used in the coping skills training. In the long-term intervention, subjects experienced more anxious preoccupation and less helplessness than the controls, but no improvement in mood or quality of life. The authors report that there were profound clinical changes in the women who attended the group, but these were not detected by the conventional measures of psychosocial adjustment.

Another psychoeducational group approach which has been intensively investigated is that of Fawzy and colleagues (Fawzy and Fawzy, 1994). From 7 to 10 patients meet for 90 minutes over a period of 6 weeks, and the group has the following four components:

1. health education

2. enhancement of illness-related problem-solving skills

3. stress management (including relaxation)

4. psychological support.

The treatment has been evaluated in patients with malignant melanoma. A total of 80 consecutive patients with stage I or II malignant melanoma (primary or local lymph node involvement) were randomly allocated to therapy or an untreated control group. Two patients were excluded from the analysis of the treatment group (one was a patient who died early in the intervention, and the other was clinically depressed). In total, 12 patients were excluded from the control group (10 individuals dropped out when they were informed that they had been assigned to the control group, and two had incomplete data). Assessments were carried out at baseline, and at 6 weeks and 6 months after the intervention. At the end of therapy the only significant difference between the groups in adjustment was on the vigour scale of the Profile of Mood States (POMS) (McNair et al, 1971). At a 6-month follow-up, the intervention group showed significantly less depression-dejection, fatigue-inertia, confusion-bewilderment, and total mood disturbance on the POMS. At the end of therapy, the intervention group reported more active-behavioural coping, and at 6 months reported more active-behavioural and active-cognitive coping than the control group. This brief treatment produced marked gains at follow-up, and also had an impact on survival (Fawzy et al, 1993) (see Chapter 4). The main methodological flaws of this study are the lack of an intention-to-treat design and the differential dropout from the two groups. In order to perform a statistical analysis it is essential that all of the participants who are randomized to a particular condition are included in the analysis. The fact that the 25% of the participants who dropped out of the control condition did not differ in terms of age, gender, degree of disease, or other demographic variables does not mean that they were identical to those who participated. It is possible that these individuals had a significant fighting spirit and would have shown an improvement in psychological adjustment through their own coping strategies over the 6-month follow-up. This would mean that those left in the control group had a poorer psychological prognosis. Fawzy et al (1996) have also compared individual treatment with group treatment, and found the group approach to be superior (see Chapter 13).

Mindfulness meditation is a development of meditation techniques used in Buddhism that has been shown to be useful in the treatment of anxiety disorders (Kabat-Zinn et al, 1992) and chronic pain (Kabat-Zinn et al, 1985). It involves learning to apply a detached awareness to moment-to-moment sensations and thoughts. Speca (1999) randomly allocated 90 people with cancer either to a 7-week group programme that taught mindfulness-based stress reduction, or to a waiting-list control. Patients in the treated group showed lower scores on the POMS for total mood disturbance, and subscales of depression, anxiety, anger, and confusion, and showed higher scores for vigour. The improvement in this sample compared very favourably with the findings of other CBT studies that have used the POMS as an outcome measure (Cunningham and Tocco, 1989; Fawzy et al, 1990a).

CBT groups

Psychoeducational groups are highly structured and didactic. Three studies have investigated the effects of more flexible cognitive behavioural interventions in a group format. Two of these (Bottomley et al, 1996; Edelman et al, 1999a,b) specifically incorporated techniques from APT.

Evans and Connis (1995) compared cognitive behavioural group therapy with supportive therapy in depressed cancer patients who were receiving radiotherapy. A total of 72 depressed cancer patients were randomly assigned to one of three conditions, namely cognitive behavioural treatment, social support, or an untreated control condition. The cognitive behavioural and social support therapies resulted in less depression, hostility, and somatization compared with the untreated control condition. The social support intervention also resulted in fewer psychiatric symptoms, and a reduction in maladaptive interpersonal sensitivity and anxiety. Both therapies also produced improvements in psychosocial function compared with no treatment, but the patients who received the social support intervention demonstrated more changes at a 6-month follow-up.

Bottomley et al (1996) reported a pilot study that compared CBT with a social support group in 31 newly diagnosed, psychologically distressed cancer patients. In total, 14 of the patients declined to have therapy and so were allocated to a decliners' non-intervention group. Nine patients received CBT and eight patients received social support. After an 8-week intervention, both groups showed limited improvement in psychological states and coping styles. The coping styles of the patients in the CBT group improved significantly compared with those of the patients in the other two groups. At a 3-month follow-up no significant differences were observed between the two intervention groups, possibly because two CBT patients had died.

Edelman et al (1999b) compared CBT and supportive therapy in women with primary breast cancer. A total of 60 women were randomly allocated to either 12 sessions of group CBT or a supportive group therapy. Both groups showed improvements in depression, quality of life, and self-esteem. However, there was significantly more improvement in quality of life and self-esteem in the CBT group compared with the supportive therapy group. The benefits of CBT over supportive therapy were no longer present at a 4-month follow-up.

Most recent studies have confirmed the efficacy of psychological interventions in improving the quality of life of patients with cancer, including CBT (Antoni et al, 2001; Kissane et al, 2003; Antoni et al, 2006), emotionally focused couple therapy (Manne et al, 2005; McLean et al, 2008), mindfulness-based stress reduction (Lengacher et al, 2009), and meaning-making intervention

(Lee et al, 2006). However, one randomized trial of supportive-expressive group therapy for women with primary breast cancer did *not* result in any reduction in emotional distress (Classen et al, 2008).

There are two main gaps in our knowledge. First, there is an absence of randomized trials that compare the different psychological therapies. The second gap concerns the quality of life of adolescent patients (Dana et al, 2009). Just four methodologically adequate studies have been published, only one of which reported a significant improvement in coping with cancer-related problems. The remaining studies found no significant changes in psychological distress and psychological functioning. Table 3.2 summarizes the results from group interventions.

Telephone therapy

Telephone therapy delivered by nurses has potential value as a way of disseminating cognitive behavioural skills. A study of older Caucasian and African American breast cancer survivors randomly allocated women to four weekly telephone sessions or usual care (Mishel et al, 2005). The intervention included audiotaped cognitive behavioural strategies for managing uncertainty about recurrence, and a self-help manual designed to help women to understand and manage the long-term side-effects of treatment. Women were taught to recognize triggers of uncertainty (places, events, or surroundings that bring back memories, feelings, or concerns about breast cancer), and then to use coping skills (relaxation, distraction, and self-talk) to manage uncertainty. The manual was a resource for dealing with fatigue, lymphoedema, pain, and other symptoms. The intervention reduced uncertainty, and the changes persisted at a 20-month follow-up (Gil et al, 2006). Doorenbos et al (2005) conducted a study of five face-to-face sessions with a nurse and five telephone sessions aimed at helping newly diagnosed patients who were undergoing chemotherapy to cope with their symptoms. The cognitive behavioural intervention was found to reduce symptom limitation. Other studies employing telephone intervention with breast cancer patients have produced only modest results (Sandgren et al, 2000; Sandgren and McCaul, 2007). This intervention consisted of six 30-minute telephone sessions delivered by oncology nurses. The patients received either breast cancer health education, sessions encouraging emotional expression, or usual care. All of the groups improved, although there was a trend which suggested that telephone therapies might relieve distress. The variability in the findings may be the result of selecting different patient groups. Alternatively, the clearer foci of the interventions used by Mishel and Doorenbos may have targeted the work in a way that the more general approach of the studies by Sandgren was unable to do.

Table 3.2 Randomized controlled trials of group CBT in people with cancer

Study	Interventions	n	Cancer type	Stage of disease	Selection	Outcome	Follow-up
Heinrich and Schag (1985)	6 sessions of stress and activity management vs. current available care	51	Commonly occurring cancers	Various stages	All patients	CBT = NTC Both groups showed improvement in psychosocial adjustment	2 months: CBT > NTC for coping in medical situations and achieving activity goals
Telch and Telch (1986)	6 sessions of group coping skills instruction vs. supportive group therapy	41	Various cancers	Various stages of disease; Karnovsky score > 70	Psychosocial distress	CBT > ST > NTC NTC group deteriorated	None
Cunningham et al (1989)	6 sessions of group psychoeducational therapy vs. supportive discussion	53	Various cancers and stages of disease	Various stages of disease	Patients referred	CBT > ST	None
Fawzy et al (1990, 1993)	6 sessions of group CBT vs. standard medical treatment	68	Malignant melanoma	Newly diagnosed	All patients	CBT > NTC	6 months: CBT > NTC
Evans and Connis (1995)	Group CBT vs. social support vs. no-treatment control	72	Various cancers	Various stages	Depressed patients undergoing chemotherapy	(CBT = ST) > NTC depression, hostility, and somatization ST > NTC Psychiatric symptoms	6 months: ST > CBT > NTC

(continued)

Table 3.2 (continued) Randomized controlled trials of group CBT in people with cancer

Study	Interventions	n	Cancer type	Stage of disease	Selection	Outcome	Follow-up
Bottomley et al (1996)	8 sessions of group CBT vs. support group vs. non-intervention	31	Various cancers	Newly diagnosed	Psychologically distressed patients	CBT = ST	3 months: CBT = ST
Edelman et al (1999)	8 sessions of group CBT vs. treatment as usual	12 4	Breast cancer	Metastatic disease		CBT > NTC Total mood and self-esteem	3 and 6 months: CBT = NTC
Edelman et al (1999)	12 sessions of group CBT vs. supportive therapy	60	Breast cancer	Newly diagnosed primary disease	All patients	CBT > ST Quality of life and self-esteem	4 months: CBT = ST
Edmonds et al (1999)	35 sessions of group support, CBT + weekend course vs. standard hospital care	66	Breast cancer	Metastatic disease	All patients	CBT + support = NTC	CBT + support = NTC
Speca et al (2000)	7 sessions of MMBSR vs. waiting-list control	90	Various cancers	Various stages	All patients	MBSR > NTC	None

Study	Intervention	N	Cancer type	Stage	Patients	Results	Follow-up
Antoni et al (2001)	10-week stress management programme vs. NTC	100	Breast cancer	Early stage	All patients	CBT > NTC, but only for depression	3 months: CBT > NTC for optimism and benefit finding
Kissane et al (2003)	20 sessions of group cognitive-existential therapy + 3 relaxation sessions vs. 3 relaxation sessions	303	Breast cancer	Early stage undergoing chemotherapy	All patients	CBT = control; trend for CBT to improve anxiety	None
Antoni et al (2006)	10-week stress management programme vs. NTC	199	Breast cancer	Early stage	All patients	CBT > NTC	1 year: CBT > NTC
Lengacher et al (2009)	6-week MMBSR programme	84	Breast cancer	Stage 0–1	All patients	MBSR > NTC for depression, anxiety, and fear of recurrence	None

ST, supportive therapy; NTC, no-treatment control; MMBSR, mindfulness meditation-based stress reduction.

Advanced disease

Until quite recently there was only evidence for the effectiveness of CBT in early-stage disease. However, trials of CBT in advanced disease are now beginning to be published. Edelman et al (1999b) demonstrated that group CBT was more effective than treatment as usual in relieving symptoms of total mood disturbance and low self-esteem in women with metastatic breast cancer. Savard et al (2006) examined the effect of cognitive therapy on women with metastatic breast cancer. A total of 45 women were randomly assigned to either individual cognitive therapy or a waiting-list control. Cognitive therapy consisted of eight weekly sessions followed by three booster sessions which were administered at 3-week intervals. The cognitive therapy group had significantly lower scores on the Hamilton Depression Rating Scale (HDRS) at the end of treatment than the control group. There was also a reduction in symptoms of anxiety, fatigue, and insomnia. These effects persisted at 3- and 6-month follow-ups.

Three recent trials suggest promising results for the application of CBT in palliative care. Greer studied 168 consecutive referrals for psychological care at St Raphael's Hospice. In total, 105 of these patients were well enough or willing to accept therapy, and were randomized to individual sessions of CBT or counselling delivered by the same therapist. The patients received an average of 6.6 sessions (range 2–14). Taking a reduction in HADS score of ≥ 2 as a sign of improvement, 76% of the CBT patients and 56% of the patients who received counselling improved. Mannix et al (2006) demonstrated that palliative care professionals could be taught basic CBT skills to use with their patients. On the basis of this, Moorey et al (2009) conducted a randomized controlled trial at St Christopher's Hospice that evaluated the effect of a training programme on the competence and clinical effectiveness of palliative care nurses who had been trained in CBT. Clinical nurse specialists were randomly allocated to receive training in CBT or to continue their usual practice. At the end of the trial, nurses were rated on the Cognitive Therapy First Aid Rating Scale (CTFARS) (Mannix et al, 2006) for CBT competence. Home care patients who scored as possible cases on the HADS entered the trial. Participants received home care nursing visits. Assessments were conducted at baseline, and at 6, 10, and 16 weeks. Eight nurses received CBT training and seven nurses continued their practice as usual. The mean CTFARS scores were 35.9 for the CBT nurses and 19.0 for the controls ($P = 0.02$). A total of 328 patients (54%) were possible cases, and 80 patients entered the trial; most of those who were excluded were too ill to participate. There was an interaction between group and time, as individuals receiving CBT had lower anxiety scores over time (coefficient = –0.20, 95% confidence interval (CI) = –0.35 to –0.05, $P = 0.01$). No effect of the training was found for depression. The trials conducted by Greer and Moorey show that it is possible to conduct a randomized trial of psychological interventions in palliative care, but that there is considerable attrition from physical morbidity and mortality.

Meta-analyses

Many of the studies described so far have suffered from the methodological drawback of small sample sizes. Meta-analysis is a statistical technique that attempts to overcome this problem by combining the results obtained from several studies. Outcome measures are converted to a common measure (the effect size) so that individual effect sizes can be pooled. The effect size is calculated from the following formula:

$$\text{Effect size} = \frac{M_1 - M_2}{SD}$$

where M_1 is the mean of the treatment group, M_2 is the mean of the control group, and SD is the pooled standard deviation for the two groups. Meyer and Mark (1995) examined 45 trials of different psychological therapies in cancer patients, and found a small mean effect size of 0.24. Sheard and Maguire (1999) criticized this study on the basis that it had included too broad a selection of trials in terms of the research questions that were asked and the outcome measures that were used. They instead chose trials which had sought to treat anxiety and/or depression. In total, 19 trials had included measures for anxiety. The overall effect size was 0.42 when treated patients were compared with untreated controls. When the 10 trials with the most reliable design were examined, the effect size was 0.36. A total of 20 trials had data on the outcome of depression. The effect size for treated patients compared with untreated controls was 0.36. There was no difference between studies that used group therapies or individual therapies. Sheard and Maguire then went on to analyse studies which had selected patients on the basis of their experiencing or being at risk of psychological distress. In these studies the impact of therapy was much more substantial. There were four trials in this category that were associated with powerful effects (Weisman and Worden, 1977; Linn et al, 1982; Telch and Telch, 1986; Greer et al, 1992). The effect sizes were 0.94 for anxiety and 0.85 for depression. These large effect sizes indicated that the average patient in the treatment conditions did better than 80% of patients in the untreated control conditions. Although the meta-analysis includes all forms of therapy, these four trials were all cognitive behavioural interventions.

This meta-analysis also revealed that group therapy was as effective as individual therapy, particularly with regard to psychoeducational courses, and that short but intensive interventions by highly trained therapists were more effective than protracted ones delivered by staff who had received less psychological training.

The authors concluded that:

> preventative psychological interventions in cancer patients may have a moderate clinical effect upon anxiety but not depression. There are indications that interventions targeted at those at risk of or suffering significant psychological distress have strong clinical effects. Evidence on the effectiveness of such targeted interventions and of the feasibility and effects of group therapy in a European context is required.

(Sheard and Maguire, 1999, p. 1770)

Akechi et al (2008) conducted a meta-analysis of six studies of patients with advanced cancer. Four of the studies used supportive psychotherapy, one used CBT and one used problem-solving therapy. The effect size for psychological treatment compared with treatment as usual was 0.44. None of the studies selected patients with clinical depression. A recent meta-analysis of CBT for depression in somatic disease (Beltman et al, 2010) found very similar results. The authors included 29 papers, of which eight studies involved people with cancer. CBT was superior to control conditions. The effect size was larger in studies of participants with depressive disorder (0.83) than in studies of participants with depressive symptoms (0.16). When the two groups were combined, the effect size was 0.49. Subgroup analyses showed that CBT was not superior to other psychotherapies.

The methodological rigour of many of the studies described here, and indeed of the meta-analyses, has been questioned (Coyne et al, 2006; Lepore and Coyne, 2006). Coyne and colleagues claim that when these trials are scrutinized they are found to show confirmatory bias and selective reporting of more favourable outcome measures. They also observe that when these trials are referred to in other papers, only the positive results are reported. These are very valid points, and the same criticism could be applied to many outcome studies in the psychosocial field. The methodology of trials is improving. For instance, trials are now being conducted with larger sample sizes and consequently greater statistical power (the average number of participants in group trials between 1990 and 2000 was 63, whereas the average number in trials conducted between 2000 and 2010 was 155). However, our hopes that therapy can improve quality of life sometimes outstrip the evidence available.

Taking all of this into consideration, it would seem that the strongest evidence is for psychosocial interventions with more distressed or symptomatic patients, and that the effectiveness of therapy with non-symptomatic patients is not established.

CBT for other common problems

Over the last 10 years, CBT protocols for specific problems have been developed and tested. The model lends itself well to this approach, which usually consists of scrutiny of cognitive and behavioural factors that might maintain the problem, generation of a maintenance model, and then construction and evaluation of a manualized intervention. We shall consider the evidence for the effectiveness of CBT for symptoms of insomnia, fatigue, and pain, and also its use as an adjuvant therapy while patients are going through a course of treatment.

Insomnia and fatigue

Sleep problems are common in people with cancer, and occur in 33–40% of patients (about twice the rate seen in the general population). Insomnia appears to be most common in lung and breast cancer (Savard and Morin, 2001; Savard et al, 2001; Davidson et al, 2002). Cognitive and behavioural techniques have a proven place in the management of insomnia in general. On the basis of the evidence available, the American Academy of Sleep Medicine (Morgenthaler et al, 2006) recommended three specific therapies for chronic insomnia, namely stimulus control, relaxation, and CBT. Smith et al (2005) reviewed the use of CBT for insomnia in patients with a range of medical conditions, including cancer, and found promising evidence of its effectiveness. A recent systematic review of psychological interventions for insomnia in cancer concluded that 'cognitive behavioral therapy interventions are likely to be effective, but effectiveness has not been established for complementary, education or information, or exercise interventions' (Berger, 2009, p. 165). A small number of randomized controlled trials have been conducted in patients with early- and later-stage disease. For instance, a recent trial compared five sessions of group CBT with treatment as usual in 150 patients who had completed active therapy for breast, prostate, colorectal, or gynaecological cancer (Espie et al, 2008). CBT had a superior effect on initial insomnia, waking during the night, and percentage of time in bed spent asleep, which persisted for 6 months.

CBT for insomnia utilizes a range of techniques that address both behavioural factors (environmental context, sleep habits, and unhelpful use of alcohol and sedatives) and cognitive factors (dysfunctional beliefs about sleep, and worry). It usually combines advice on sleep hygiene with changing sleep-related behaviours and evaluating unhelpful thinking (Smith and Neubauer, 2003). We shall discuss how these techniques can be applied within a standard course of APT in Chapter 11. Improvement in sleep following CBT appears to be associated with changes in dysfunctional beliefs about sleep, and a reduction in daytime naps (Tremblay et al, 2009).

There is a strong association between sleep and cancer-related fatigue, although the causal relationship, if any, has yet to be clarified (Zee and Ancoli-Israel, 2009). Up to 90% of people with cancer experience fatigue, making this the most frequently reported symptom associated with cancer and its treatment (Lawrence et al, 2004; Hofmana et al, 2007). A recent review by Kangas et al (2008) identified 57 randomized controlled trials that employed either physical exercise or psychological interventions to improve cancer-related fatigue. There were no significant differences between the two types of intervention (the effect size for psychological treatment was 0.31 and that for physical exercise was 0.41). The authors commented that multimodal exercise and walking programmes, restorative approaches, and supportive-expressive and cognitive behavioural psychosocial interventions showed promise. None of these studies specifically selected patients with clinically significant levels of fatigue so, as with many studies of anxiety and depression, there could well be a floor effect. The results also suggest that vigour and vitality respond to interventions independently from fatigue. A recent study compared a brief nursing intervention aimed at enhancing physical activity with CBT, and found CBT to be more effective (Goedendorp et al, 2010). The effect of CBT did not appear to be mediated through an increase in physical activity.

Pain

One-third of people with cancer experience pain, and three-quarters of people with advanced cancer have pain. Furthermore, 12–51% of patients with cancer report that they do not have adequate pain control (Larue et al, 1995; Zech et al, 1995) There is now sufficient evidence for the effectiveness of CBT in pain management for it to be given the highest level of evidence rating in guidelines for managing cancer pain (Cormie et al, 2008; Scottish Intercollegiate Guidelines Network, 2008). Pain management is often delivered in groups with a psychoeducational format and modules including education, relaxation, exercise training, goal setting (Robb et al, 2006), and problem solving (Sherwood et al, 2005). Tatrow and Montgomery (2006) conducted a meta-analysis of CBT techniques for distress and pain in breast cancer patients, and found effect sizes of d = 0.31 for distress ($P < 0.05$) and 0.49 for pain ($P < 0.05$), indicating that 62% and 69% of breast cancer patients receiving CBT had less distress and less pain, respectively, relative to the control conditions. There were larger effect sizes for individual treatment compared with group treatment for distress, but not for pain. The correlation between effect sizes for distress and pain was not significant, which suggests that the interventions had a differential impact on the different symptoms. The idea that tailoring interventions to specific aspects of the patient's pain is more effective in reducing pain than a more general, non-specific form of CBT is supported by a study by Dalton et al (2004). They compared standard CBT with a treatment based on patients' responses to the Biobehavioral Pain Profile (BPP) (Dalton et al, 1994) in patients with a mixture of cancer diagnoses, targeting techniques at environmental influences, loss of control, healthcare avoidance, past and current experience, physiological responsivity, and thoughts of disease progression. Compared with standard CBT, pain profile-tailored CBT had a greater effect on current pain, average pain, and overall quality of life.

Conclusions

There is compelling evidence from randomized controlled trials that CBT can significantly improve the quality of life of patients with primary and advanced cancer who are emotionally distressed. In our trial, these effects had persisted at a 1-year follow-up.

◆ There is some evidence that other psychological therapies (such as supportive-expressive therapy, meaning-based therapy, and emotionally focused therapy) benefit patients' quality of life. Studies comparing CBT with other therapies have so far been inconclusive.

◆ Individual and group therapies appear to be equally effective. In clinical practice, patients express strong preferences for one approach or the other. Therefore both therapies should be made available.

◆ The effect of psychological intervention on unselected, non-distressed cancer patients is minimal, and it is therefore not recommended in this patient group.

◆ There is a dearth of information about the effect of CBT and other psychological therapies on the quality of life of adolescent cancer patients.

Chapter 4

Can psychological therapy affect duration of survival?

In an astonishing clinical report that was published in 1848, John Elliotson, a British physician, claimed that he had successfully treated a woman with cancer of the right breast ('scirrhus cancer') by means of hypnosis conducted for five years. During that period, the tumour shrank and then disappeared completely. Elliotson's report is of historical interest only. The vast majority of the medical profession, including the present authors, have always assumed that the course of cancer cannot be influenced by any psychological intervention. However, this assumption was challenged in 1989 by Spiegel and his colleagues in their landmark study of women with metastatic breast cancer. Their randomized clinical trial revealed that patients who received group therapy ($n = 50$) survived for an average of 18.9 months longer than patients in the control group ($n = 36$) who did not receive group therapy (Spiegel et al, 1989).

'Supportive-expressive' group therapy was conducted weekly for at least 1 year. According to Spiegel (1985), this therapy had four components. First, patients were encouraged to express their feelings and fears about their illness. They encouraged each other to be assertive and to recognize and express anger in appropriate ways. Anxiety about death and dying was addressed directly. Secondly, physical symptoms were addressed – for example, by teaching the women how to control their experience of pain by means of self-hypnosis and relaxation. Thirdly, mutual support figured prominently during therapy. Fourthly, issues concerning the meaning of life were explored, as patients reassessed their life values, focusing on projects that were still possible during the remainder of their lives. Spiegel observed that the sense of extracting meaning from tragedy was an important aspect of therapy.

It is not surprising that Spiegel's study created enormous interest. For the first time, a randomized controlled investigation had demonstrated that psychological intervention – in this case, supportive-expressive group therapy for a period of 1 year – had a significant favourable effect on survival of patients with metastatic cancer. This finding was completely unexpected, as the study had been designed to determine the effect of group therapy on mood disturbance (Classen et al, 1998). Spiegel and his colleagues looked for other possible explanations for their finding by testing 26 variables (including age, initial staging, number of days of irradiation, type of surgery, time interval between initial diagnosis and death, and degree of metastatic spread) for baseline differences between the therapy and control groups that could account for the difference in duration of survival. None of these variables explained the difference in survival. Having exhausted other possibilities, the authors drew the logical conclusion that the difference in survival time was due to group therapy. Strenuous efforts to refute this conclusion have been made by Fox (1998a). He argues that the survival curve for patients in the control group appeared to be unusually steep. When compared with that of a population with metastatic cancer from the same region, the control patients who survived for longer than 20 months were 'an extremely aberrant sample subject to the strong biasing influence of possible confounders, of which a considerable number are known, but not including those accounted for in the study.' His criticisms were answered in detail by Spiegel et al (1998). This was followed by a rejoinder from Fox 1998b), which in turn produced strong arguments against Fox's views from Goodwin et al (1999) and Speca (1999), followed by yet another rejoinder by Fox (1999). The debate highlights the formidable problems that are encountered in this particular area of research. Readers with an interest in methodology will find the debate informative.

A number of studies followed Spiegel's original trial. Richardson et al (1990) studied 94 patients with various haematological cancers. Patients were randomly assigned either to one of three treatment conditions or to a control group. The treatment conditions consisted of an educational programme and a home visit, or the same educational programme plus 'shaping', or the educational programme plus 'shaping' plus a home visit. The educational programme was delivered by a trained nurse who described in detail the disease and its treatment, emphasizing the importance of compliance with treatment, and persuading family members to ensure that the patient took the prescribed drugs. 'Shaping' involved the nurse working with the patient so that the latter learned to take responsibility for self-medication. At follow-up 2 to 5 years later, the patients in all of the educational intervention groups had an improved survival rate compared with the patients in the control group. This finding was maintained after differences in treatment compliance had been taken into account.

Of particular interest is the investigation of 68 patients with stage I and II malignant melanoma, in a study conducted by Fawzy et al (1990a,b, 1993). Their psychological intervention consisted of six weekly sessions of group therapy which were focused on health education, stress management, coping skills, and group support. Patients were randomly allocated to either the support group or a control group. Their outcome measures included immune responses and psychological responses up to 6 months after the psychological intervention, and survival 5 to 6 years later. With regard to immune responses, psychological intervention was associated with a significant increase in the percentage of natural killer cells, in natural killer cell activity, and in CD8 (suppressor/cytotoxic) T cells. Higher levels of natural killer cell activity predicted survival. Psychological intervention significantly reduced depression, fatigue, and mood disturbance, and enhanced coping skills. At a 6-year follow-up, patients in the control group had a significantly higher death rate (10 out of 34 patients) than those who had received the psychological intervention (3 out of 24 patients). Fawzy and Fawzy (1994) concluded that 'psychiatric interventions that enhance effective coping and reduce affective distress appear to have beneficial effects on survival.'

Each of the studies considered so far has reported significant associations between duration of survival and either group therapy (Spiegel et al, 1989; Fawzy et al, 1990a,b, 1993) or an educational programme (Richardson et al, 1990). However, there are other psychological intervention studies which have not found any effect on survival. In the first of these studies, Linn et al (1990) examined the effect of individual supportive psychotherapy on 120 men with various metastatic cancers (predominantly lung cancer). Therapy focused on encouraging patients to express their feelings, to exert personal control (where possible) in their lives, and to find some meaning in their lives. Patients were randomly allocated to either a therapy group or a control group. At follow-up 1 year later, duration of survival was similar in both groups. A second study with negative results was reported by Ilnyckyj et al (1994). A sample consisting of 127 patients with a variety of cancers at various disease stages was studied. Patients were randomly assigned either to a control group or to one of three psychological intervention groups. Psychological therapy consisted of weekly sessions of group therapy for 6 months. One group was led by a social worker, another group was led by a social worker for 3 months and then 'peer led', and the third group was entirely 'peer led.' It is not clear what kind of group therapy was given. At follow-up 11 years later, duration of survival was found to be similar among patients in the control and therapy groups. It should be noted that this study lacks information concerning the nature of the psychological interventions.

Another investigation to be considered here is a randomized controlled trial of group therapy by Cunningham et al (1998), who studied women with metastatic breast cancer. In total, 30 patients received 35 weekly sessions of supportive plus cognitive behavioural therapy. The control group consisted of 36 patients who received only a home-study cognitive behavioural package.

At a 5-year follow-up, the authors found no significant difference in survival between the therapy and control groups. However, it should be noted that the numbers were small, and may have been insufficient to reveal a difference in survival. Furthermore, the control group was not an untreated group, as patients in this group used relaxation audio tapes, and 28% of them attended an external support group. There is therefore some doubt about these negative results. The authors themselves state that 'our clinical impression, in agreement with that of many who have long experience of psychological work with cancer patients ... is that some patients, particularly those who become very involved in trying to help themselves, do much better than is expected medically.'

A study of group CBT for patients with metastatic breast cancer was conducted by Edelman and her colleagues (Edelman et al, 1999a,b). A total of 124 patients were randomly allocated to either CBT or a standard care control group. Three patients were subsequently found not to have metastatic disease, and were therefore excluded from the study. Data for known medical prognostic factors were obtained. CBT consisted of a core programme of eight weekly sessions and a 'family night', followed by three further monthly sessions. Patients were taught a range of cognitive and behavioural strategies, such as thought monitoring, cognitive restructuring, and goal setting, as well as completing homework exercises. Statistical analysis of 121 patients entered in the study at a 2- to 5-year follow-up revealed that there was no survival advantage associated with CBT.

Replication of the studies of Spiegel and Fawzy

Two replication studies of Spiegel's original trial failed to confirm his findings (Classen et al, 1996; Goodwin et al, 1996). A further randomized trial of supportive-expressive therapy in women with metastatic breast cancer reported that therapy did not prolong survival but did improve quality of life (Kissane et al, 2007). A very well-designed replication of Fawzy's study also failed to show any effects on survival (Boesen et al, 2005).

However, a subsequent randomized trial of psychological intervention in women with regional but non-metastatic breast cancer revealed that a reduced risk of recurrence and death among the patients was associated with psychological intervention (Andersen et al, 2008). Psychological intervention was undertaken in small groups, and consisted of strategies to reduce stress, improve mood, alter health behaviours, and maintain adherence to cancer treatment. The reduced risk of recurrence and of death, although statistically significant, was modest. At an 11-year median follow-up, 75 women who had received psychological intervention were free of disease, compared with 65 women in the control group ($P = 0.016$). The median duration of survival was 6.1 years for women who received intervention, compared with 4.8 years among controls.

One other study reported positive results. Kuchler et al (2007) conducted a randomized trial of psychotherapeutic support in patients with a preliminary diagnosis of cancers of the oesophagus, stomach, liver, gallbladder, pancreas, colon, and rectum. Individual psychotherapy was provided, which consisted of ongoing emotional and cognitive support to foster fighting spirit and reduce helplessness and hopelessness. At a 10-year follow-up, a statistically significant improvement in survival was found among patients who received individual psychotherapeutic support compared with patients who received standard care only ($\chi^2 = 11.73$, $P = 0.006$). These results applied to patients with stomach, pancreatic, primary liver and colorectal cancer.

In the most recent trial (Ross et al, 2009), patients with colorectal cancer (70% Dukes' stages B and C, 14% with distant metastases) were randomized to psychosocial intervention or treatment as usual. Psychosocial intervention consisted of between one and ten home visits by a nurse or medical doctor who provided information and emotional support. There was no systematic psychotherapy. Follow-up at 2 years revealed no effect of this kind of psychological intervention on survival.

There have been criticisms of methodology directed specifically at trials revealing positive results (Coyne and Palmer, 2007). Although some of their criticisms may be pertinent, their final conclusion is certainly not. Coyne et al (2009) have commented that 'It is reasonable to expect that areas of investigation that have failed the tests of science be denied financial support. After all we do not fund work on phlogiston theory, astrology, or crystal therapy.' To compare the effect of psychotherapy on survival to these discredited topics is grossly unfair and misleading. More important still, to proscribe the present area of research is unscientific. As Kraemer et al (2009) have pointed out, 'Good science answers questions and questions answers, but it does not declare certain questions off limits.'

Is randomization appropriate?

Cunningham et al (1998) have put forward an interesting suggestion. In their experience, relatively few patients make the kind of substantial psychological changes (in lifestyle, attitudes, awareness of mind–body connections, and other factors) that could influence their physiology sufficiently to affect duration of survival. Such highly motivated people tend not to be common or available for randomized group assignment. They are individuals who take steps to get the therapy that they want. Therefore, if only a small proportion of the patients who are undergoing psychological intervention make significant changes, the effects may be lost when group medians are calculated and compared, unless the number of subjects is very large. In addition, the distribution of such highly motivated patients in small experimental groups may be strongly influenced by chance. Cunningham argues that, instead of randomization, a different kind of experimental design is more appropriate, namely single case studies in which individuals are followed up over a period of years, and changes in their psychological functioning are compared with the extent to which these patients outlive their predicted survival according to medical prognostic features.

These are persuasive arguments. There may well be a place for single case studies in which the patient is their own control (Aldridge, 1992). However, a major weakness of single case studies is that one cannot make valid generalizations as is the case with randomized studies. Admittedly, randomized controlled trials have certain limitations. Ethical problems arise in deciding whether and when it is justified to compare a new treatment with current treatment or with no active treatment. There are often considerable difficulties in explaining randomization to patients and obtaining genuine informed consent. Large numbers of patients are required in order to ensure, as far as possible, that the experimental and control groups are similar in all respects except for the treatment under investigation. Moreover, the results of randomized trials are based on comparisons between group means, and do not tell us whether any given individual patient will benefit from psychological intervention. In the words of one critic, 'randomization tends to obscure rather than illuminate interactive effects between treatments and personal characteristics' (Weinstein, 1974). On the other hand, there can be no doubt that prospective controlled trials are essential if we are to avoid or minimize the influence of bias. Randomization is not the only way to attempt to avoid bias. Matching is another option, but randomizing to experimental and control groups is regarded by most investigators as the most effective and bias-free methodology (Bradford Hill, 1961; Cawley, 1983; Fox, 1998a; Spiegel et al, 1998). For this reason, we have considered only randomized controlled studies in this review. As we have noted, randomization has its problems. However, in the absence of a demonstrably superior method of eliminating bias we are stuck with it. Winston Churchill once described democracy as the worst form of government except all the others that have been tried. Similarly, randomization could be regarded as the least unsatisfactory method of dealing with bias.

Summary and conclusions

The studies cited in this chapter were randomized trials, and biological prognostic factors were taken into account when determining the effect of psychological therapy on survival. The inconsistent results from trials involving patients with different cancers, different stages of cancer, and different psychological interventions preclude any definitive conclusions. However, some tentative conclusions, which are subject to possible revision in the light of future trials, may be offered.

1. Neither supportive-expressive nor cognitive behavioural group therapy appears to have an effect on survival in women with metastatic breast cancer.

2. Women with less advanced (i.e. non-metastatic) breast cancer may survive longer when given psychological therapy in small groups. This encouraging result needs to be verified in replication studies.

3. Insufficient numbers of trials involving patients with cancers other than breast cancer have been published to warrant any conclusion.

4. In view of the overwhelming influence of biological factors on the course of cancers, it is unlikely that psychological therapy can affect the duration of survival in patients with metastatic or other advanced cancers. The majority of the published trials bear out this conclusion.

5. Psychological therapy may result in a modest improvement in the duration of survival of patients with non-metastatic breast cancer. However, verification is needed from further large carefully controlled trials.

Part Two

CBT for People with Cancer

Chapter 5

Overview of therapy

The place of psychological treatment in oncology

Since the last edition of this book was published, the field of psychosocial oncology has continued to grow, and the need for psychological support has been recognized in official guidance. In 2002 we proposed the following three levels of expertise and intervention:

1. basic skills among health professionals, including breaking bad news, identifying and managing distress, providing information, and recognizing problems that require intervention from a more specialist service

2. provision of interventions within oncology services, including counselling or other psychological interventions in the form of brief informal therapy or longer-term support as part of the work of nurse specialists or social workers

3. specialist psycho-oncology services delivered by liaison nurses or liaison psychiatrists.

The National Institute for Clinical Excellence (2004) has recommended that a four-tier model of professional psychological assessment and intervention should be implemented in each Cancer Network in the UK, according to the *Supportive and Palliative Care Improving Outcomes Guidance*. Health and social care professionals should be responsible for providing support at levels 1 and 2, while more severe psychological distress (levels 3 and 4) should be managed by a variety of psychological specialists. These include counsellors, mental health nurses, clinical and health psychologists, psychotherapists, and liaison psychiatrists. There is recognition that specialists may need to work across the Cancer Network, in primary care and the community as well as in hospitals and hospices. All professionals who are working with cancer patients should be able to recognize psychological needs and be skilled in listening, giving effective information, communicating compassionately, and delivering general psychological support (level 1). Some staff will be trained further in identifying psychological distress and using simple psychological interventions such as problem solving (level 2). At the next level (level 3) some professionals will deliver counselling and specific psychological interventions, such as anxiety management and solution-focused therapy, according to an explicit theoretical framework. Mental health professionals will deliver level 4 care, which consists of specialist psychological and psychiatric interventions, including CBT. The availability of these services is still very variable. There are initiatives for training oncology professionals in basic communication and psychological intervention skills, with some encouraging evidence for the usefulness of these skills (Mannix et al, 2006; Moorey et al, 2009). Access to mental health professionals is often more difficult, and they may not always have sufficient confidence to work with people with life-threatening illness.

CBT can be applied across all four levels of psychological support. At levels 1 and 2 we have successfully helped nurses in palliative care to formulate psychological distress within a cognitive framework, and to employ basic cognitive and behavioural techniques (Cort et al, 2009). Sage et al (2008) have published a workbook and toolkit that provide a helpful CBT resource for oncology professionals. This volume is aimed more at professionals with some mental health or CBT training who wish to learn how to apply these skills for people with cancer (levels 3 and 4), although many of the concepts and interventions are applicable to levels 1 and 2.

We originally called this form of CBT 'adjuvant psychological therapy' (APT). Just as one might expect to receive adjuvant chemotherapy, it should be equally acceptable to receive adjuvant psychological therapy (Cunningham, 1995). APT is therefore designed to be used alongside and as an aid to physical forms of treatment in an integrated treatment setting. With its emphasis on fostering a positive attitude, helping the patient to collaborate with and cope with treatment, and reducing emotional distress, this therapy can complement traditional medical treatment. Some of the theoretical and clinical components can be used at all four levels. For instance, when a patient is considering whether or not to go ahead with a course of chemotherapy, an oncologist could collaboratively help the patient to assess the costs and benefits of the treatment (see Chapter 9). Cognitive behavioural techniques can be used more formally by specialist breast care nurses or Macmillan nurses in a group or individual format. Clinical psychologists and psychiatrists will find this therapy particularly applicable to the more distressed patients who are referred to them.

This therapy is intended for use across a broad spectrum of problems, ranging from people with no abnormal symptoms who want help to enable them to cope better with cancer, to those with definable psychiatric illness. However, the majority of patients will access this therapy because they are experiencing distress. People who are undergoing *adjustment reactions* constitute the largest group that is referred for psychological treatment. With these patients more emphasis may be placed on non-directive techniques in the first instance, facilitating the expression of negative emotions before moving on to the problem-solving components of therapy. With *mild to moderate depression* or *anxiety*, APT looks very much like standard CBT. Ventilation may be less important, particularly if there is a well-established chronic maladaptive adjustment style. The National Institute for Health and Clinical Excellence (NICE) guidelines on the treatment and management of adults with chronic physical health problems recommend that CBT should be available for moderate depression (National Institute for Health and Clinical Excellence, 2009). *Relationship problems* and *sexual problems* associated with cancer can also be addressed using this approach, but in relationships that have a history of long-standing conflict or disturbance, the impact of cancer is often of secondary importance. A brief focused therapy that is aimed primarily at improving personal and marital adjustment to physical disease may be unsuitable, and these couples may require formal marital or family therapy. There are well-established cognitive behavioural approaches to these problems which can be applied to people with cancer (Beck, 1988; Dattilio and Padesky, 1990; Dattilio, 1997; Jacobson et al, 2000; Shadish and Baldwin, 2005).

Anticipatory nausea occurs in up to 10% of patients who are treated with chemotherapy (Aapro et al, 2005). Nausea and anxiety are experienced shortly before receiving chemotherapy, and may be triggered by specific environmental cues, such as syringes, white coats, or hospitals. This condition responds very well to a combination of cognitive and behavioural treatments (Watson and Marvell, 1992; Watson, 1993), and it has been demonstrated that the treatment methods can be used by health professionals who do not have extensive psychological therapy training (Morrow et al, 1992).

Cancer pain can also be alleviated with cognitive behavioural techniques (Turk and Fernandez, 1991; Crichton and Moorey, 2002).

APT is not suitable for patients who are *actively psychotic*. The cognitive behavioural techniques that have been applied successfully in schizophrenia (Kuipers et al, 1997; Kingdon and Turkington, 2005) require special training and experience. This does not mean that patients with a diagnosis of schizophrenia who are in remission, or whose psychotic symptoms are reasonably well controlled, cannot benefit from therapy. The same proviso applies to patients with *organic psychoses*, such as confusional states or dementia. It is important to work closely with the oncologists who are treating the patient to ensure that any organic causes of psychological reactions have been investigated

Table 5.1 Psychological disturbances encountered in oncology, and guidelines for the application of APT

Suitability for APT	Disorder
Suitable	Adjustment reactions
	Depression
	Anxiety
	Sexual problems
	Relationship problems
	Anticipatory nausea
	Pain
Possibly suitable (may require modified treatment, e.g. combination with drug therapy, or longer duration of treatment)	Severe depression
	Severe anxiety
	Coexisting personality disorder
	Alcohol abuse
	Major pre-existing relationship problems
Unsuitable	*Active psychoses*
	Schizophrenia
	Bipolar affective disorder
	Organic psychoses
	Confusional states
	Dementia

and treated before embarking on a course of therapy. People with *more severe forms of depression or anxiety states* will often require a combination of psychotherapy and pharmacological treatment as recommended by the NICE guidelines (National Institute for Health and Clinical Excellence, 2009).

The majority of patients with adjustment reactions can be treated with APT in the form described in this book. Table 5.1 summarizes the types of psychological disturbance that are encountered in oncology, and gives guidelines for the use of APT with each condition.

The theoretical basis of APT

The cognitive model of adjustment (see Chapter 2) proposes that it is the appraisals, interpretations, and evaluations that the individual makes about cancer that determine his or her emotional and behavioural reactions. It is not the symptoms of the disease or the effects of treatment per se that produce the emotional response, but rather the meanings they hold for the person involved. How the individual thinks about the illness and its implications for their life is central to adjustment. If the predominant meaning of cancer is loss, the person will feel depressed. If cancer represents a potential threat to health, security, or life itself, the emotional response will be one of anxiety. However, if the person perceives the disease as an intrusion into and unjust violation of their world, their reaction will be one of anger. Adjustment involves an interpretation of the type of stress that cancer imposes, evaluation of how well the stress can be managed, and the mobilization of coping behaviours. Emotional reactions will obviously vary as the disease itself changes or the person seeks different ways to interpret their situation.

As we saw in Chapter 2, everyone has a set of basic assumptions about themselves and their world, which do not usually include beliefs that they will develop cancer. One of the tasks for the individual with cancer is to make sense of the diagnosis, either by incorporating the experience into their world view, or by modifying their beliefs. Some authorities insist that cancer makes people modify their beliefs by realizing that the world is not benevolent (Janoff-Bulman, 1999). Others point to the way that an individual can manage to retain 'positive illusions' – for instance, by emphasising that there are other people who are worse off, even in the face of serious illness (Taylor et al, 2000).

After an initial period of turmoil, most patients develop a relatively stable *adjustment style* (see Box 5.1). The most significant threat that cancer poses is to the very survival of the patient. There are five common adjustment styles (see Chapter 2), and each represents a slightly different way of viewing the threat to survival. These form a constellation of thoughts, feelings, and behaviours which the individual uses to enable them to cope. The individual adjustment style can be seen as a *cognitive schema*. It is like a template that makes sense of the disease, its treatment, the individual's response, and the future outcome. People with maladaptive adjustment styles tend to have a rigid schema. There is a cognitive triad which involves a negative view of the diagnosis, control of the disease, and its prognosis. For instance, the patient with a helpless/hopeless response perceives the diagnosis as a death sentence, believes that

Box 5.1 Common adjustment styles

Fighting spirit

Denial

Fatalism

Helplessness/hopelessness

Anxious preoccupation

there is nothing anyone can do about it, and feels hopeless about the future. Information about cancer is processed in a biased fashion. *Cognitive distortions* maintain the helpless/hopeless schema by filtering out hopeful information while magnifying negative information about the disease. Patients will over-generalize from a single event ('I felt too ill to do much today; I'll never be able to do the things I want to do'), or they may think in a black and white fashion ('If I can't do everything I used to do, there's no point in doing anything'). The more entrenched the maladaptive adjustment style, the more negative is the thinking. These patients have frequent *negative automatic thoughts* which may be very unrealistic and exaggerated. Such thoughts maintain the patient's emotional distress and prevent them from using effective coping strategies. Other modes of adjustment operate in a similar way (see Table 5.2). There is obviously a spectrum ranging from realistic to unrealistic thoughts and atti-tudes about the disease, and for many people with advanced disease a pessi-mistic view of their prognosis is correct, but maladaptive adjustment styles distort reality to make it even bleaker than it really is. The helpless/hopeless patient with advanced disease will focus on their inability to do anything about the disease or their quality of life, instead of looking at ways in which the dis-ease can be controlled and the quality of remaining life can be enhanced.

The meaning of cancer and the threat of death are probably the most impor-tant factors that influence patients' adjustment. However, for some people other factors related to the disease may be of more significance. There may be

Table 5.2 Patients' perceptions of diagnosis, degree of personal control, and prognosis in different adjustment styles

Survival schema			
Adjustment style	**Diagnosis**	**Control**	**Prognosis**
Fighting spirit	Challenge	Believes that he or she can control the disease and/or life	Good
Denial	Minimal threat	Irrelevant	Good
Fatalism	Minimal or major threat	Believes that others can control the situation, but that the patient him- or herself cannot	Unknown
Helplessness/ hopelessness	Major threat, loss or defeat	Believes that nothing can affect the disease outcome	Poor
Anxious preoccupation	Major threat	Is uncertain about his or her ability to exert control over the disease	Uncertain

a realistic belief about the possibility of recovery, but the side-effects of treatment may seem intolerable.

Some patients are distressed by the effects of surgery, and if the emotional upset that they experience is severe or prolonged it will require help. There are often negative automatic thoughts that reflect unrealistic self-deprecation. For example, patients may think 'I'm hideous, I can't go out like this', or 'No one could possibly love me.' For others it may be the effects of the disease on significant areas of their life that cause problems. Many men consider themselves less worthy if they have to give up employment as a result of cancer. These factors usually imply some kind of threat to the person's self-image through loss of attractiveness, loss of role, loss of self-esteem, etc. Prior to developing cancer, individuals generally have a fairly stable view of themselves in relation to other people and the world. This can be seen as a *self-schema* which integrates memories, beliefs, and goals related to the self-image. Cancer does not necessarily impinge upon this. However, in some cases the effects of cancer or its treatment may become a major threat to the self. For instance, if a person has a strong belief that they can only be happy if others find them attractive, any disfigurement as a result of treatment can seriously damage their self-esteem. Patients who experience difficulty in coping may develop a negative image of themselves as ugly, diseased, or unlovable. Patients who experience a threat to their usual self-image will experience intense anxiety – for example, if a woman believes that chemotherapy will make her bald and unattractive. These two areas of threat, namely *threat to survival* and *threat to the self*, may exist separately or together, and the cognitive structures that are involved interact.

If this survival schema becomes more generalized, it can apply to areas of the patient's life that are unrelated to cancer. A helpless/hopeless response can turn into depression as negative thinking becomes generalized to views about the self, the world, and the future unrelated to the disease. An anxious preoccupation can generalize to become an anxiety state. In developing a stable adjustment style, patients often go through many different interpretations of their situation. Feelings of anger, sadness, and fear are a normal part of this adjustment process. It may be that a certain degree of emotional processing is necessary in order to develop an adaptive way of coping with the disease. Patients who avoid these emotions, or who do not have a supportive social network in which to express them, may encounter difficulties in adapting to the disease.

The final component of the theory behind CBT for people with cancer concerns the interactive nature of coping with cancer. The disease occurs in a social context, and important people in the patient's life will influence his or her feelings. Friends, relatives, and health professionals will all provide informational and emotional support. The way that the patient interprets the behaviour of these individuals will contribute to the emotional response that is observed. For example, a woman with breast cancer believed that the reactions of her friends to news of her illness would be a mixture of pity and gossip, so she decided not to tell anyone about her diagnosis. Another woman with ovarian cancer discovered that telling people about her diagnosis brought her a sense of relief and also a feeling of self-confidence that she could reveal this, even if her friends' reactions were less supportive than she had hoped.

The patient's partner plays a very important role in the patient's ability to cope. The dynamics of the relationship can often be dramatically affected by cancer. Suppression of emotions, particularly anger, can lead to communication problems between the patient and their partner which require psychological help.

From this theoretical framework it is possible to generate the aims of therapy.

Aims of therapy

These are as follows:

1. to reduce emotional distress
2. to improve mental adjustment to cancer by inducing a positive fighting spirit
3. to promote in the patient a sense of personal control over their life and active participation in the treatment of their cancer
4. to develop effective coping strategies for dealing with cancer-related problems
5. to improve communication between the patient and their partner
6. to encourage open expression of feelings, particularly anger and other negative feelings, in a safe environment.

Format of therapy

APT developed as a modification of Beck's cognitive therapy. Experience in treating people with cancer at King's College Hospital and the Royal Marsden Hospital, London generated a number of practical strategies for dealing with the problems encountered by this group of patients. This clinical experience has been used to adapt the cognitive therapy methods that are traditionally employed with patients suffering from states of anxiety and depression. APT is delivered over 6 to 12 weekly sessions, each session lasting for 1 hour. Therapy is problem-oriented, and the problems encountered may be emotional (e.g. depression), interpersonal (e.g. problems in communicating with the partner), or related to the cancer type (e.g. body image problems in mastectomy patients). The patient is taught the cognitive model of adjustment to cancer and shown how their thoughts contribute to their distress. This educational component is important, as it provides the rationale for the coping strategies that the patient learns during therapy. Each therapy session is structured by setting an agenda to deal with one or more of these problems. Regular homework assignments are used to give the patient experience of finding alternative, more constructive ways of thinking, and of developing new coping strategies.

The therapeutic relationship is one of 'collaborative empiricism', whereby the patient is taught to examine their beliefs about cancer, and to treat them as hypotheses which can be tested. If someone has early-stage disease with a good prognosis, a statement such as 'I know I'll be dead by next year' is tested by considering the evidence for and against it. Often beliefs are based upon misconceptions, or upon no evidence at all. Even when cancer is more advanced, such a thought may be overly pessimistic, because it assumes an inevitable certainty about the course of the disease. The therapist also collaborates with the patient to find and employ strategies for coping with cancer. Therapy is conceptualized as a joint problem-solving exercise, where the insights and suggestions of the patient and their partner can be as useful as those of the therapist.

Components of therapy

Emotional expression

Although emotional expression is unlikely to be therapeutic if it is the sole procedure in a therapy, it can have an important place as part of treatment for patients who are undergoing adjustment reactions. Ventilation of feelings is often needed before a problem-solving approach can be used. Anger appears to be one emotion which people with cancer find hard to express (Watson et al, 1984), and APT therefore sets out to facilitate the constructive expression of anger (see Chapter 7).

Behavioural techniques

Behavioural techniques are usually employed in the early stages of therapy. The techniques are the same as those used in CBT for anxiety and depression, including graded task assignments and activity scheduling, behavioural experiments, relaxation, and distraction. Cancer robs patients of control of their own bodies, and its treatment involves more passivity than the treatment of other conditions. This loss of control can generalize to other areas of the patient's life. Behavioural techniques help to give a sense of mastery or control over the patient's life and environment. Behavioural assignments can help the patient to develop a sense of control over the disease itself by encouraging cooperation with treatment or the use of self-help techniques such as visualization. They can also develop control in areas unrelated to cancer, and indirectly foster a fighting spirit.

Cognitive techniques

During the session the therapist elicits automatic thoughts associated with the problems that the patient is facing, and shows the patient how to identify their own negative thoughts. From the first or second session the patient is set the task of monitoring their thoughts between sessions. Once these cognitions can be recognized, the next step is to learn to test them. A variety of techniques can be used for this process of cognitive restructuring. *Reality testing* involves examining the evidence for a particular thought or belief. This allows realistic, sad, or anxious thoughts to be distinguished from distorted negative thinking. A technique that can be used for distressing realistic thoughts as well as unrealistic ones is the *search for alternatives.* Here the patient is encouraged to explore all of the possible explanations, predictions, or ways of looking at something to see if more realistic or more positive alternatives are available. *Decatastrophizing* encourages the patient to think about what they fear, to see if it is really that bad. For instance, a patient who is terrified of recurrence can consider what treatment might be available and what methods of fighting the disease they might develop if it did recur. Testing the *effect of negative thinking* helps to show that even when a thought is realistic, it is not necessarily helpful, because it may interfere with the person's ability to problem solve or to get on with their life. When the patient can recognize these negative automatic thoughts, more realistic or more constructive thoughts are used as responses. Often the cognitive change will suggest a *behavioural plan* that can help to consolidate the new way of thinking. If the patient is less convinced that the alternative way of thinking is that appropriate, they can try *behavioural experiments* to test the old and new beliefs.

Working with couples

There are two main ways in which partners are involved in APT. They can act as powerful co-therapists, reminding the patient of their strengths, remembering times when they have coped effectively in the past, and providing reinforcement for successful coping efforts. Relationship problems are addressed using a combination of cognitive and behavioural techniques, with a strong emphasis on facilitating communication.

The following chapters will describe the techniques in more detail. Because APT uses behavioural, cognitive, emotion-focused, and interpersonal techniques, it can be described as a multimodal therapy (see Box 5.2). The techniques are

Box 5.2 Characteristics of APT

Based on a cognitive model of adjustment to cancer

Structured

Short term (6 to 12 sessions)

Focused and problem oriented

Educational (the patient is taught coping strategies)

Collaborative

Makes use of homework assignments

Uses a variety of treatment techniques:
- non-directive methods
- behavioural techniques
- cognitive techniques
- interpersonal techniques

tailored to the particular needs of the individual. Some patients do not have a partner, so individual therapy is the only method available. Some individuals need to spend a lot of time just talking about their feelings, whereas others can move into a problem-solving mode straight away. Many patients make rapid gains with behavioural techniques alone, and do not take to cognitive techniques, while others do not show any behavioural deficits, so cognitive interventions are the major therapeutic method.

Phases of therapy

This flexible approach means that aims and techniques are changed and developed over the course of therapy in response to the patient's needs. It is not possible to lay down hard and fast rules about the course of therapy. However, it is sometimes useful to consider the treatment as three broad phases. These phases usually have slightly different aims, and different techniques are emphasized as a result.

Beginning therapy

The aims of the initial stage of therapy are as follows:

1. *Symptom relief*: the therapist works with the patient to develop coping strategies for immediate problems. The latter will usually involve either emotional distress, such as depression and anxiety, or life crises.

Problem-solving and behavioural techniques such as distraction, relaxation, graded task assignment, and activity scheduling are used during this phase.

2. *Living an ordinary life:* the therapist explains the principles of maximizing the quality of life available. The patient and their partner are helped to plan as active and rewarding a time together as is possible within the constraints of the disease. The daily activity schedule is used as a basis for this. Activity scheduling helps to:

   • build on strengths
   • use mastery and pleasure experiences to promote control
   • encourage the patient and their partner to plan new goals.

3. *Teaching the cognitive model:* aims (1) and (2) above should be met within a cognitive framework. As problems are defined and addressed they are formulated in cognitive terms. The therapist repeatedly uses examples from the patient's thoughts and feelings. With some individuals it may be possible to begin thought monitoring during this stage.

4. *Encouraging the open expression of feelings:* the patient is encouraged to express and accept negative emotions such as anger and despair before they are subjected to any reality testing. *The art of APT lies in achieving the right balance between facing the fears of cancer and positively avoiding them through the active approach described in aim (2) above.*

The length of this phase will depend on the client's response. It will usually last for two to four sessions.

Middle stage of therapy

By the end of the first stage the patient's emotional distress should have been relieved to some extent, and they should be familiar with the cognitive model. The middle phase of therapy continues this work within a more explicitly cognitive framework. The aims of this phase are as follows:

1. *Teaching the use of thought monitoring and the basic principles of dealing with unhelpful thinking:* the Dysfunctional Thoughts Record (DTR) is used as a regular self-help assignment.

2. *Continuing the process of problem solving:* the focus gradually shifts from the priorities of the first stage (i.e. reducing emotional distress and dealing with life crises) to less urgent but equally important issues (e.g. social isolation, communication problems between the patient and their partner, difficulty in coping with the unpredictability of cancer). The patient and their partner adopt an increasingly active role in problem solving as therapy progresses.

3. *Continuing the process of fighting cancer:* Improving quality of life is still a goal, but now cognitive techniques are added to the behavioural techniques. Some patients may wish to explore ways in which they themselves can take active steps to improve their prognosis.

This stage lasts for three to six sessions.

Ending therapy

By the end of the middle stage, the patient and their partner have learned new ways of engaging in life and countering negative thoughts. Not all of the problems may be completely resolved, but the couple will have the means to continue the process beyond therapy. The final stage looks to the future in the following ways:

1. *Relapse prevention:* coping strategies are discussed which can be used in the future if the cancer recurs, or if other stresses in the person's life threaten to cause emotional disturbance. With selected patients, discussion of cancer recurrence and death may be appropriate.

2. *Planning for the future:* as therapy progresses, provided the prognosis is reasonably good, more long-term goals can be discussed. Couples are encouraged to set up realistic goals to be achieved in 3, 6, or 12 months' time, and to come up with practical plans for achieving them.

3. *Identifying underlying assumptions and core beliefs:* for some individuals it may be appropriate to look at the beliefs that give rise to their emotional problems, and to help them to change some of the rules that they habitually apply to themselves and to the world. Many people want to change their lifestyle as a result of their encounter with cancer (e.g. by placing less emphasis on work-related achievement, living more healthily, etc.). These positive changes can be discussed at this stage if appropriate.

This stage can last for one to three sessions. The extent to which these issues are covered in detail will depend on the person's response to the previous phases of APT.

Illustration of APT

The following case demonstrates some of the basic principles of APT that have been outlined in this chapter. To make the illustration of the techniques clearer, a case has been chosen which involved mainly individual therapy. Case descriptions elsewhere in the book will show how APT is used with couples.

Susan was a 34-year-old woman with breast cancer who was treated with excision biopsy followed by radiotherapy. Two years later a recurrence was discovered in the same breast, with metastatic nodes in the other breast. She was reluctant to have a mastectomy or to undergo chemotherapy, and was started on tamoxifen. As the size of the tumour increased despite hormone treatment, Susan eventually agreed to chemotherapy, receiving three courses of different combination therapies without improvement. She became anxious about the effects of further treatment on her appearance, particularly fearing the loss of her hair. She felt increasingly irritable, depressed, and lethargic, and asked to be referred for psychological help. At interview she had a mildly depressed mood, with symptoms of loss of motivation and pleasure, indecisiveness, and ruminations about cancer. In particular she was preoccupied with the effects of cancer on her appearance. A diagnosis of mild reactive depression with anxiety was made. Therapy consisted of 12 weekly sessions of APT. Susan was seen with her husband for the first session, but he was only able to attend on one other occasion, despite attempts to engage him.

Beginning therapy

Problems identified in the first session were as follows:

1. depressed mood
2. preoccupation with loss of attractiveness, and mistrust of her husband
3. marital conflict.

One of the first goals was relief of Susan's depressed mood. She remarked that 'It's just as if everything I've planned I haven't been able to do … why plan anything?' The therapist encouraged her to express her feelings of anger and hopelessness. While showing empathy for her sadness over the very real losses caused by cancer, the therapist challenged the absolute nature of these statements. These negative thoughts and Susan's loss of motivation became the focus for helping her to concentrate on living an ordinary life. The therapist challenged her belief that there was no point in doing anything by getting her to identify things that she was still able to plan. Activities were found which still gave her pleasure, and realistic goals were set as homework for the next week (e.g. buying Christmas presents and going out with a friend). She was thus able to gain control over some ordinary areas of her life that had not been affected by cancer. Negative automatic thoughts such as the one described above were elicited early in therapy and used to demonstrate the cognitive model. Activity scheduling continued over the first four sessions, and this helped to increase Susan's mood and motivation.

Middle stage of therapy

In subsequent sessions Susan learned how to identify automatic thoughts herself. She began to monitor automatic thoughts on occasions when she felt depressed or anxious. For instance, while she was in a supermarket one day with her husband, he joked with a shop assistant. She immediately thought 'He's flirting with her. What a cheek! What does he get up to when I'm not with him?' This made her feel insecure and deserted. Her negative thoughts then continued: 'He's going to leave me eventually. I might as well leave him first.' On examination it seemed that she had been sensitized to rejection by the experience of her husband getting cold feet before their wedding, but subsequently he had been supportive and shown no signs of wanting to leave. She could not remember any time since their marriage when he had flirted with anyone. She was encouraged to continue this process of reality testing and to substitute more realistic thoughts when she started worrying that he was going to leave. During this part of therapy she continued the process of trying to live a normal life, and she found it useful to make concrete plans on a weekly basis.

Ending therapy

Towards the end of therapy the assumption underlying Susan's negative thoughts was discovered. She believed that she could only be of value if she was sexually attractive. She was encouraged to examine whether attractiveness really referred solely to physical appearance, or whether it might apply to other characteristics. She was helped by the idea that it was only part of her body which looked different, and in fact in her daily life she looked no different from usual because she had not suffered any major side-effects from chemotherapy. She found that her mood improved as a result of APT, while there was some reduction in her need to base her self-esteem solely on her physical appearance.

Practical considerations

The following chapters will consider the methods and format of CBT for people with cancer in more detail. Before we move on to the techniques, it may be helpful to cover some of the practical matters that need to be taken into account when embarking on a course of therapy. Table 5.1 summarizes the problems that are suitable for therapy, together with those conditions for which APT is contraindicated. Beyond this it is difficult to say who is most likely to benefit from treatment. Patients with early disease and a relatively good prognosis may well respond best, as these individuals can test their negative thoughts about cancer against the touchstone of a realistically good future. However, this does not mean that patients with advanced disease cannot do well. Our experience is that many people have been effective copers, and then decompensate when they face advanced or terminal illness. A brief cognitive behavioural intervention can often help them to regain their confidence and coping abilities, with dramatic results. Studies of CBT in advanced cancer have shown promising results (Savard et al, 2006; Moorey et al, 2009). Fighting spirit in these cases means optimizing the quality of life, as in the case of Susan, rather than looking forward to cure.

APT is usually given over 6 to 12 sessions. Many patients do well with the shorter course of treatment, but some require the full 12 sessions. When considering taking therapy beyond 6 sessions, the degree to which the patient's symptoms have been relieved should be taken into account, together with the extent to which the patient and their partner have learned the principles and techniques of APT. Early symptom improvements in the absence of any evidence that coping strategies have been learned may lead to recurrence of psychological distress. When cancer activates core negative beliefs about the self and the world that are derived from early life experiences, it may not be possible to produce major changes within just a few sessions. Therapy then needs to be extended for a longer period, and much of the work involves understanding how beliefs that the world is a dangerous and abusive place arose, and how cancer confirmed these beliefs, so that less destructive views can be explored and acted upon.

Chapter 6

The therapy session

Although the therapist–patient relationship and the structure of therapy are often referred to as non-specific aspects of treatment, they are actually essential to the successful use of more specific interventions. This chapter will show how both are necessary for effective CBT.

Important aspects of the therapeutic relationship that are covered include the following:

♦ warmth, genuineness, and empathy from the therapist

♦ the fostering of a partnership to test thoughts and beliefs (collaborative empiricism)

♦ the use of guided discovery to question thoughts and beliefs.

CBT puts more emphasis on structuring sessions than other therapies. In this chapter we shall discuss the following:

♦ how to structure the first session, including establishing rapport, defining problems and goals, explaining the model, and setting the first homework

♦ how to structure subsequent sessions

♦ the basic principles of agenda setting

♦ the value of frequent summarizing

♦ the importance of eliciting feedback.

The therapeutic relationship

The same basic interpersonal skills are needed in CBT as in any other form of psychotherapy. The patient needs to feel that he or she is understood. An interested, committed therapist will be more appreciated than an aloof one. If a good therapeutic relationship does not exist, techniques such as challenging negative thoughts may appear confrontational and cold. It is therefore vital that the technology does not hinder the relationship between patient and therapist.

The role of warmth, genuineness, and empathy in psychotherapy has been intensively investigated. It accounts for 7–10% of the variance in therapy outcome (Bohart et al, 2002). Cognitive behaviour therapists regard these factors as important but not exclusively significant in producing change. People with cancer need to feel that their therapist has understood something of what they have been going through, and that he or she is genuinely interested in them as people and in their well-being. Burns and Auerbach (1996) reviewed the role of therapeutic empathy in CBT, and concluded that the effects of therapeutic empathy on recovery from depression are large 'even in a highly technical form of therapy such as cognitive therapy.' A working alliance in which the patient trusts the therapist and is prepared to discuss and explore painful thoughts and feelings is very important in therapy. Although it is easy to see when a therapist has achieved this kind of rapport, it is more difficult to specify what behaviours are needed to achieve it. Thwaites and Bennett-Levy (2007) have divided therapeutic empathy into four components, namely empathic attunement, empathic attitude/stance, empathic communication, and empathy knowledge.

Many of the techniques described in Chapter 7 can aid the development of rapport. CBT fosters a therapeutic relationship in which the patient and the therapist are partners in problem solving. Two essential components of this partnership are *collaborative empiricism* and *guided discovery*.

Collaborative empiricism

Beck coined this term to describe the special relationship that develops in cognitive therapy. Therapy is empirical because it is constantly setting up and testing hypotheses. It is collaborative because the patient is actively involved in this process, helping to define problems and devise solutions both inside and outside the session. There are distinct advantages to this approach. By using the empirical model, the patient's negative *beliefs* are turned into *hypotheses* which can then be tested.

A belief that a patient cannot regain their old sense of control over their life becomes a prediction that they will not be able to overcome feelings of helplessness:

'I can understand that at the moment it seems you will never be able to get back to your old self after everything you have been through. I know of many people who have been able to make something of their lives in these circumstances, but you may well be different from them. Since neither of us can foretell the future, perhaps we could test out your beliefs by trying an experiment. Would you be willing to try some of the things that other people have found useful in overcoming their feelings of helplessness?'

A belief that the cancer might come back at any time and therefore must be guarded against at all costs can be reframed as a prediction that checking for signs of recurrence every day is the best coping strategy:

'At the moment you are checking that the cancer hasn't come back every day. You say that doing this helps to reassure you as well as make sure you pick up a recurrence as soon as possible. Perhaps we could examine whether all the checking you are doing is as helpful as it seems.'

Collaborative empiricism allows the therapist to acknowledge that the patient's view of the world makes sense. Giving up if everything seems hopeless, or checking if they fear secondary spread, are both perfectly sensible behaviours within the patient's belief systems. Rather than taking the belief at face value, the therapist helps the patient to look for evidence of its accuracy and usefulness. Some people take well to this model. Therapy then becomes a truly collaborative venture, in which the patient can be as creative as the therapist in devising methods of coping.

Guided discovery

One of the best methods for helping someone to test their thoughts and beliefs is through guided discovery. Asking questions to clarify what the person believes and what evidence there is to support that belief is a much more acceptable and effective way to change attitudes than persuasion. Many negative thoughts about cancer are true, while others may be distorted or unhelpful. Asking questions enables the patient to separate the realistic thoughts from the unrealistic ones without giving the impression that all negative thoughts are somehow 'wrong.' When working with life-threatening illness it is always better to adopt a stance of inquiry rather than disputation. Guided discovery should lead the patient to ask whether there might be an alternative, more constructive view of the situation which could help them to fight cancer better. It alternates questions with empathic statements that summarize the person's thoughts and feelings, and should help the patient to synthesize all of the information about the problem into the most adaptive evaluation. Here is an example of how guided discovery can be used with a patient who is feeling helpless:

Therapist: What makes you think there's no point in trying?

Patient: It just seems never-ending, I've seen all those other patients coming back again.

Therapist: Does anything in particular go through your mind when you see that happen?

Patient: Yes, I keep thinking I'll be just the same.

Therapist: That must be a horrible feeling, just the inevitability of it.

Patient: Yes, that's how it feels – inevitable.

Therapist: Did the people you are thinking of have the same type of cancer as you?

Patient: Yes, one of them did.

Therapist: Do you know anyone else who had your type of cancer, but didn't go through many hospital admissions?

Patient: Well, perhaps one or two.

Therapist: Do you think more about the people who did well or about the person who had lots of admissions?

Patient: I think a lot more about the person who just kept going into hospital again and again. I know I shouldn't, but I just can't help it.

Therapist: What effect does that have?

Patient: It makes me feel even worse.

Therapist: Even more hopeless, as if it really is inevitable?

Patient: Exactly.

Therapist: So you think more about the person who had a rough time, which makes you feel worse, and you sort of assume that you're going to have the same experience. Is that assumption based on anything you know about your own disease, or is it based more on the *feeling* you get when you remember your friend?

Patient: I suppose it's the feeling really. I don't have any reason to believe my illness has to go the same way as hers.

Therapist: What do you make of that?

Patient: Well, it looks as if I'm assuming that because it *feels* that way it's going to *be* that way. It might not be as inevitable as it seems.

The use of questioning is an important component of all of the cognitive techniques that will be described later.

The structure of APT

Beck's cognitive therapy has a number of structural elements that have been found to be helpful in brief psychotherapy with emotionally distressed patients (Beck, 1995). APT incorporates these structural elements in the treatment programme for cancer patients. Before looking at how a typical therapy session is structured, we shall consider the first session. In this session there are some special requirements. The patient (and their partner) must be engaged, the problems must be elicited, the rationale of APT must be explained, and the business of therapy begun.

The first session

Since much CBT in liaison settings is brief, the first meeting with the patient is very important in getting therapy started on the right footing. We describe an approach to treatment that combines assessment and the start of treatment at the first meeting. This has certain advantages, as it allows the business of learning to cope with problems to be started straight away. The first session may last from 60 to 90 minutes. This method does not suit all clinicians, and some prefer to carry out a full and detailed assessment before instituting any therapy. Both of these approaches are compatible with APT. We here describe how to use the first session as a therapeutic session. Several goals need to be accomplished during this first session.

Establishing rapport

Most people who are referred for psychological help in oncology have not had any previous contact with psychiatry or psychotherapy. It is therefore vital that they are engaged during the first session, or they may not return. The best way to establish rapport is through the use of non-directive counselling techniques and the demonstration of empathy. Listening, reflecting back the patient's statements, and summarizing them succinctly all contribute to the feeling of being understood. As we have said, the fact that APT is a directive, problem-oriented therapy does not lessen the importance of these non-specific factors. They are probably more important than in other cognitive behavioural therapies, because of the relief that patients under stress obtain as a result of expressing their feelings. It is usually helpful to begin by asking the patient to tell something about the way the cancer was discovered, and the history of treatment, and to cover relevant aspects of the person's life history. This approach both gathers information and builds rapport by showing an interest in the patient as a person.

Rapport is also established through pursuit of the other goals of the first session. Defining problems helps the patient to feel less overwhelmed, and this establishes the therapist's credibility, while explaining the rationale of APT gives the patient and their partner a framework within which to understand the problems.

Defining problems and goals

As the patient expresses their feelings about the experience of cancer, the therapist can help to reframe these as a focus for therapy. The starting point must always be the patient's and partner's own perceptions of the problems that they are facing. These may be symptoms such as depression, anxiety, or irritability, or life problems such as financial difficulties, the stage the disease has reached, etc.

In the first interview the couple's thoughts and feelings about the disease should be explored, as well as the implications of cancer for the patient's self-image.

Information from the following assessment instruments may be helpful in this process of problem formulation.

1. *The Hospital Anxiety and Depression Scale* (HADS) (Zigmond and Snaith, 1983) is a 14-item measure of mood which was designed for use with patients with physical illness. Seven items measure anxiety and seven items measure depression. Its psychometric properties have been investigated in cancer patients (Moorey et al, 1991). This scale provides information about the severity of emotional symptoms (cut-off scores of 8 for depression and 10 for anxiety indicate clinical cases), and responses to individual questions can point to problems to be targeted.

2. *The Mental Adjustment to Cancer Scale* (MACS) (Watson et al, 1988) measures styles of adjustment to cancer. The MACS has five subscales (fighting spirit, helplessness-hopelessness, anxious preoccupation, fatalism, and positive avoidance), which provide information about the adjustment style that the patient is using.

3. *The Cancer Coping Questionnaire* (CCQ) is a 21-item questionnaire designed at the Royal Marsden Hospital to assess the cognitive, behavioural, and interpersonal coping strategies that are taught in APT. Its reliability and validity have been recently investigated (Moorey et al, unpublished manuscript). Patients' responses to individual questions can provide information about their coping strengths and deficits.

4. *The Cancer Concerns Checklist* (Harrison et al, 1994) assesses 14 cancer concerns. Patients who have four or more concerns, or who have concerns about sexuality, feeling upset, or feeling different are more likely to suffer from anxiety or depression. Responses to this measure can be used as a starting point for discussion of target problems.

These assessment questionnaires are reproduced in Appendix 5.

Typical problems that might be identified include the following:

1. General problems unrelated to cancer type (e.g. feelings of helplessness, the unpredictability of the outcome, fears of death and recurrence, treatment).

2. Specific problems related to cancer type (e.g. feeling dirty with regard to cancer of the cervix or the bowel, feeling unfeminine with regard to cancer of the breast, or worries about sexuality, which are more common in breast, gynaecological, and testicular cancers).

3. Emotional disturbance (e.g. depression, anxiety, guilt, anger).

4. Interpersonal problems (e.g. arguments with partner, social isolation, feeling different).

5. Physical problems (e.g. lethargy, nausea, pain, inability to do things).

6. Socio-economic problems (e.g. work-related problems, financial difficulties).

It is not possible to exhaustively explore every problem, but by the end of the session a list of the most important ones can be drawn up. This exercise in problem definition is the first step in showing the patient that they can regain control over some aspects of their life. Once the list has been drawn up, the therapist can collaborate with the patient and their partner in choosing the problems that are most important. When doing this, account should be taken of the issues that the couple consider to be a priority. The therapist should also look for problems that can be tackled quickly and effectively. For example, a patient may say that her greatest problem is knowing what decisions to make about her child's future. If the patient is depressed, this may be too big an issue to deal with early in therapy. It may be better to accept the importance of this problem, but to leave it until later, focusing initially on other symptoms such as depressed mood, lack of interest, or hopelessness. When the woman's mood has improved she will feel more able to think about making major decisions.

A 40-year-old woman with carcinoma of the ovary was referred because, although she had an encapsulated tumour which was caught very early, she had great difficulty in accepting that her prognosis was good. During the interview she described feeling very hopeless, frequently tearful, and tense. She was sure that the cancer was still there, and was constantly thinking about how it might have spread elsewhere in her body. This was not helped by the fact that she had recently had a liver scan for what was initially thought to be a metastasis, but in fact proved to be a benign cyst.

In addition to the cancer, she described other stresses in her life. Her boyfriend was unable to make a firm commitment to the relationship, her 15-year-old daughter was behaving rebelliously, and she was under extreme pressure in her job as a lecturer. She appeared very anxious during the interview, and was fidgety and spoke rapidly.

The therapist took a background history, but focused on this patient's current problems. A problem list was drawn up (see Table 6.1).

The therapist was sensitive to the patient's feeling of being under great pressure, and helped her to conceptualize her anxiety symptoms as a response to the stresses she was experiencing as a result of cancer and her life situation. The first intervention consisted of teaching her anxiety management techniques involving relaxation and the identification of anxiety-provoking thoughts. This focus allowed the therapist to teach the patient coping strategies that could be applied to the various problem areas. Later on in therapy these areas were addressed in their own right.

It is often possible to move from the problem list to goals during the first session. Questions such as 'How would you know that this problem had been solved/reduced?', 'What would need to happen for this problem to be less

Table 6.1 Patient's problem list

Problem	Goal
Anxiety and stress	Learn strategies for dealing with anxiety and stress
Attitude to cancer – hopelessness and anxious preoccupation	Become more hopeful, and get through a week without being preoccupied with cancer
Relationship with boyfriend	Short-term goal: Enjoy time with boyfriend without pressuring him Longer-term goal: Make decisions about the relationship
Relationship with daughter	Be able to spend 2 hours together each week where we have quality time and don't argue
Stresses at work	Manage my workload so that I feel I am on top of the demands that are being made of me

worrying?', and 'Can you think of something that you will be able to do when this problem has been alleviated?' elicit realistic, attainable, and wherever possible behaviourally defined goals.

Explaining the cognitive model and rationale of therapy

In a short-term therapy, much of the emphasis is placed on developing skills that the patient can continue to use after therapy has ended. In order to use these self-help skills properly, the patient must understand their rationale. The basic features of APT are explained in the first session. Automatic thoughts are elicited, and the therapist shows the patient how these thoughts contribute to their emotional distress. The patient will not understand the concepts fully in the first session, but usually they are able to grasp the idea that their thoughts may in some way be contributing to their distress. It is essential that the therapist introduces the key concepts of cognitive therapy: *the way we view situations determines our reactions to them.* Three main points are explained.

1. APT is active, directive, and aimed at helping the patient to develop a constructive and positive approach to coping with cancer.

2. APT is based on cognitive therapy. Examples from the patient's own experience are used to show the relationship between thoughts and feelings.

3. The practicalities (e.g. 6 to 12 sessions, joint meetings, use of self-help assignments) are explained.

The educational process continues throughout therapy. The patient needs to understand the purpose of each new intervention, whether it is behavioural or cognitive, and to see how it might be applied in other situations. We shall consider how the rationale for various techniques can be explained to the patient when we cover those interventions in succeeding chapters of this book.

The importance of providing some sort of road map for therapy cannot be underestimated. Fennell and Teasdale (1987), using Beck' cognitive therapy with depressed patients, have found that acceptance of the cognitive model predicts response to therapy. They were able to divide patients who received cognitive therapy into rapid and slow responders. Those who responded rapidly were more likely to react positively to the explanation of the cognitive model of depression in the first session, and were also more likely to have a positive response to the first homework assignment. The rationale provides a framework in which the patient and their partner can understand their reactions to cancer, and it also offers hope. Patients benefit from reading the booklet *Coping with Cancer* (see Appendix 1). This will usually form part of the first homework assignment, and is used to reinforce the educational component of the first session.

The cognitive model at this stage will usually only cover the interaction between the patient's thoughts, feelings, mood, and behaviour, and will demonstrate how the current problems relate to these systems. Drawing a diagram of this interaction may be very helpful for both therapist and patient. In some cases a deeper conceptualization is possible even from the first session. The individual's core beliefs might emerge as very obvious themes from the problem list and history.

Setting homework

In addition to asking the patient to read *Coping with Cancer*, the therapist will usually set a homework task designed to address one of the patient's presenting problems. This will most often be a behavioural task, but may sometimes be a cognitive assignment, such as the monitoring of negative thoughts. Anxious patients can be taught relaxation and then asked to practise this over the following week. Depressed patients often benefit from some structured tasks, such as scheduling of pleasant activities, or activities that induce a sense of personal control. In the examples cited above, the woman who had an anxious preoccupation with her ovarian cancer was given two homework tasks. First, she was asked to record her experience of stress over the following week in whatever circumstances this occurred. The therapist drew up a chart for her that included sections on degree of stress, the situation in which it occurred, and automatic thoughts associated with it (see Table 6.2). The second task was to listen to a relaxation tape and if possible to practise some relaxation exercises each day. In addition, the woman read *Coping with Cancer*.

Table 6.2 Monitoring stressful situations: first homework assignment

Situation	Stress rating (0–10)	Automatic thoughts	Coping response
Boyfriend not arriving on time	7	He wants me to think he is finishing with me. He shouldn't put me under all this stress	Busied myself Watched television
Daughter ate the crisps I was keeping for a party	9	My God, I can't keep anything in the house. She ought to help me more She's not thinking of me	Drank two glasses of sherry Yelled at her to get it out of my system

Not all patients will be able to follow such a demanding programme. This woman was intelligent and well educated, and she very quickly grasped the requirements of therapy. For other patients, particularly those with more disabling symptoms, expectations may be more modest. Performing a simple task such as visiting a relative may be all that some patients can be expected to do after the first session.

The structure of subsequent sessions

After the first or second session the format settles down to a regular pattern. Feedback from the previous session, the events of the last week, and the success or failure of homework assignments all need to be covered, as well as the main problem that the patient wishes to discuss. The usual plan for a therapy session can be summarized as follows:

1. Set the agenda. Only one or two topics should be included.
2. Review the patient's week and obtain feedback from the previous session.
3. Review the patient's homework. Identify the main details (e.g. lessons learned or difficulties experienced).
4. Start on the main topic of the session.
   (a) Define the problem clearly.
   (b) Identify associated negative thinking.
   (c) Answer this.
   (d) Work out how to handle the problem differently in the future.
5. Set the patient's homework. Make it relevant both to the individual and to the content of the session.
6. Ask for feedback.

Although the structure of the sessions remains constant, the content will vary depending on the phase of therapy and the nature of the problems that are being experienced by the patient and their partner.

Agenda setting

Because APT is a short-term therapy, time is at a premium. The structure of the session allows time to be used effectively by agreeing an agenda with the patient and summarizing particular issues and interventions during the session. The structure of therapy allows flexibility and is not applied rigidly, but rather it serves as a framework. Sometimes it may be necessary to step outside this framework. For instance, if the patient has recently been told of a recurrence of the disease and needs to express their feelings immediately, it may be inappropriate to set a formal agenda. However, by the end of the session, when the patient has ventilated their feelings, it is usually possible to reassert the structure by summarizing the content of the session and looking for coping strategies that the patient might try out.

At the beginning of each session the patient and the therapist decide on the main topics for discussion. Part of the agenda will consist of feedback on the last session, a report on the patient's homework, and a brief review of the previous week. The rest of the session is then devoted to the main agenda items. It is usually best to limit these to only one or two items. It is also helpful, after starting work on a problem, to continue with that problem at the next session so that significant inroads are made into it, rather than switching from one problem to another. Once an agenda has been set, it is best to adhere to it unless a very important new item (e.g. suicidal ideation) arises which needs to replace it.

The advantages of agenda setting are as follows:

1. It allows judicious use of the short time available.
2. It helps to model the process of problem definition and problem solving.
3. The structure that is provided helps to keep the patient on track. This is particularly important in the case of patients whose attention and concentration are impaired by depression or anxiety.
4. If it is used well, the patient contributes to agenda setting as part of the collaborative relationship.

Summaries

The therapist makes summaries several times during the course of a session of CBT, usually after an important intervention or at the end of an agenda item. This helps to clarify both for the therapist and for the patient what the cognitive conceptualization of the problem is and what methods have been developed to deal with it. A final summary at the end of the session is also useful. Summaries help to keep the patient and the therapist on track, and aid the retention of insights and therapeutic strategies. As therapy progresses, the patient becomes increasingly responsible for providing these summaries. This is another way of empowering the patient and finding out how much learning has occurred during the session.

A typical capsule summary might be as follows:

From what we have been discussing today it seems that attractiveness is an important issue for you. We began by looking at situations which make you feel bad, and found that they often involve meeting other women. When we examined the thoughts you had in these situations, they all had the theme of comparison. You said 'She's prettier than me' or 'I hate her – *she* hasn't had a mastectomy.' The next step is to see whether these thoughts and comparisons are realistic and helpful. Before we do that, could you tell me whether I've summarized the problem correctly?

Feedback

A therapeutic alliance can only be established if the professional has a clear idea about the client's perception of the problem, the therapy, and the therapist. Surprisingly, traditional psychotherapy has not paid much attention to gathering information systematically about the patient's reactions to particular interventions in therapy. CBT makes use of regular feedback, both at the end of each session and at strategic points during the session. Asking for feedback also helps to prevent difficulties in the therapeutic relationship. On the whole, transference is not a focus in this type of therapy, so wherever possible collaborative therapeutic relationship is encouraged so that a problem-solving approach prevails. Distorted thoughts about the therapist or therapy can hinder this.

For example, a woman who had been treated for malignant melanoma 12 months previously had developed an anxious preoccupation with the disease. Although there were no signs of recurrence, she could think of nothing else. During the first session she initially showed immense relief at being able to talk about her anxieties to a sympathetic listener. The therapist gradually led her to the point where he asked about her fears of death, of which she spoke reluctantly. Later on in the session she changed her attitude dramatically and asserted that she was all right now and would get better. When the therapist tried to talk about some strategies for managing her anxiety, the patient became very angry. After the therapist asked her for feedback on his effect on her, it emerged that she had perceived the questions as being too negative. She only wanted to hear good things about cancer, and believed that the therapist was acting wrongly in apparently forcing her to think about her fears. This problem might have been prevented if the therapist had been more sensitive to her emotional change during the session, and had asked for feedback earlier.

Feedback frequently reveals that the patient and the therapist have very different ideas of what was useful in the session, which is a salutary finding. Feedback also reveals stumbling blocks to between-session assignments. Automatic thoughts such as 'I'll never do it', 'What's the point?' or 'It won't work' are common responses to homework assignments, but the patient often only expresses these thoughts if specifically asked about them. Once such thoughts have been identified, they can be challenged within the collaborative relationship.

Summary

In CBT, as with all psychotherapies, the personal skills of the therapist form the basis upon which a therapeutic relationship is established. Skills in listening, reflecting, and showing empathy are used in everyday life, and some people find it easier to use them than others. In addition to these basic skills, CBT fosters a particular type of relationship that involves collaboration in solving problems, where the therapist helps the patient to test beliefs through a process of guided discovery. This collaborative empiricism allows the patient and their partner to develop their skills as 'personal scientists.' The collaborative relationship is embedded in a structured therapy session that uses agenda setting, summaries, and regular feedback to maximize the alliance between patient and therapist in learning new skills for coping with cancer. Whether the techniques employed are cognitive, behavioural, or emotive, the structured collaborative therapy session is a hallmark of CBT.

Chapter 7

Experiencing and expressing emotions in adjuvant psychological therapy

As we have seen in the first part of this book, learning that one has a potentially fatal illness can shatter one's assumptions about one's world and oneself. Reconstructing one's world view requires both cognitive and emotional processing, yet at times the sheer enormity of the threat and the raw emotions that are experienced can be overwhelming. Horowitz (1986) postulated two oscillating phases in the adjustment process, namely 'overmodulated' emotions where avoidance and denial are manifested, and 'undermodulated' emotions where overwhelming feelings are experienced. The person who is facing a trauma moves between these emotional states as the system tries to regulate affect so that the new information can be incorporated into old schemas, or new schemas can be formed. The behavioural and cognitive techniques described in Chapters 8, 9, and 10 are mainly aimed at helping the patient to regulate undermodulated negative emotions. In this chapter we shall discuss how emotions can be shut down or overmodulated when the impact of cancer becomes too threatening. The mechanisms of avoidance of emotional experiencing will be described, and also the way that people often try to suppress strong feelings. The importance of acknowledging and expressing emotions in the adjustment process will be considered.

We shall describe the following clinical skills:

◆ when to facilitate emotions and when to help the patient to regulate them
◆ how to facilitate emotional experiencing and emotional expression
◆ working with denial
◆ methods for helping the patient to ventilate and channel anger.

Avoidance of negative emotions

From a cognitive perspective, three different processes may operate to prevent an individual from experiencing strong emotions in the face of objectively distressing events. These are cognitive distortion, cognitive avoidance, and affective avoidance.

We have already introduced the concept of *cognitive distortion* in its negative form (see Chapter 5), and we have also talked of our tendency to operate a slight positive bias. For instance, Weinstein demonstrated that people overestimate the likelihood of experiencing positive outcomes in life and underestimate the likelihood of experiencing negative events (Weinstein and Lachendro, 1982). This positive bias may shift imperceptibly from an optimistic view (which we call fighting spirit) to an objectively unrealistic optimism (which we call denial). Many people with cancer persist in thinking that they will be cured against all the odds. They may deny that their illness is life-threatening. In extreme cases they may even deny that they have cancer at all. As we described in Chapter 2, this denial can be regarded as a negative schema that makes sense of the cancer and the threat to survival. Cognitive distortion minimizes the impact of the disease. In denial, cognitive distortion operates in an unrealistically positive way, while in the other adjustment styles the distortions are usually negative. The consequence of attending exclusively to the good news one hears and excluding the bad news is that one reduces the perceived threat and so avoids having to experience painful emotions.

We encountered an example of this positive distortion when testing a coping measure in our research some years ago. A 60-year-old woman with cancer of the cervix had undergone a radical vulvectomy. She had a colostomy and urostomy, but despite all of this she appeared very cheerful. She scored low on the Cancer Coping Questionnaire because she did not feel in the least stressed and did not believe that there were any problems with which she needed to cope. She did not consider that her operations had caused any difficulties in her life at all, and reported spontaneously how she had been very amused when her grandson had said 'You're very lucky, granny, you can go to the toilet and go shopping all at the same time.' This woman was selectively filtering out all of the negative aspects of her disease. She did not see it as a challenge or threat, but only as a minor irritant.

A second way to avoid painful feelings is to focus attention elsewhere. *Cognitive avoidance* occurs when an individual voluntarily or automatically avoids thoughts and images that might cause distress. This process is used by all of us at times (e.g. focusing on other topics, distracting ourselves, saying 'It's best not to think about it'), and it can be an adaptive coping strategy. At other times it is only partially effective and the negative emotions break through, but the patient does not have immediate access to the cognitions that produce the feelings. An example of this might be a man with cancer of the larynx who cries inexplicably while watching television. He may have no idea why he feels so upset. Further probing of the situation might reveal that he was watching a programme in which a man argued with his wife and shouted at her. This reminded him of how difficult he found communicating strong emotions after undergoing a laryngectomy. Cognitions such as 'I can't have a good row any more' or 'I can't get across how I feel' may have occurred at the time, but he rapidly avoided them.

The final form of avoidance, namely *affective avoidance*, is a dissociative mechanism in which the person blocks off the painful emotions. The patient is able to talk about distressing events without any emotional reaction. This may sometimes protect them from painful feelings, but often this dissociation may be associated with somatic symptoms such as headaches, dizziness, etc. The woman who had a vulvectomy was practising affective avoidance when she discussed realistically the effects of her operation, but did not have any associated feelings.

Positively biasing perception and interpretation, distracting oneself from painful thoughts, and dissociating from painful emotions are all forms of experiential avoidance, which has been defined as 'the reluctance to remain in contact with experiences such as feelings, thoughts, and bodily sensations, and attempts to alter, control, predict, or avoid the form, the frequency or the contexts in which these experiences arise' (Fledderus et al, 2010, p. 504). In the adjustment phase it may be helpful to shut down when feelings become too overpowering, and to gradually titrate how much one exposes oneself to aversive experiences. They are part of the overmodulation of affect necessary in the emotional processing of traumatic events. However, in the longer term experiential avoidance may be unhelpful, because attempts to control what one is thinking or feeling may actually increase the intrusiveness of the very experiences that one is trying to escape (Gold and Wegner, 1995).

Suppression and expression of negative emotions

Many people experience appropriate negative emotions but do not express them openly. There are several factors that make acknowledging and expressing emotions difficult for a patient with cancer. The patient's position is one of relative helplessness, making it difficult for them to show anger or 'fight' in the sick role. Fears of abandonment by professionals, relatives, or friends if they are perceived as difficult or 'bolshy' can prevent the patient from showing how scared or angry they really feel. Motives such as altruism (i.e. selflessness based on concern that caregivers should not be burdened with negative emotions as they have so much to cope with already) can also contribute to emotional suppression in this situation. For a long time there has been a clinical impression that people with cancer appear to suppress their emotions, and that they are more likely to subjugate their own needs to those of other people. There is some support for this impression. Fernandez-Ballesteros et al (1998) compared 311 women with breast cancer with 103 healthy women. Women with breast cancer had higher scores on 'anti-emotionality' as measured by the Rationality/Emotional Defensiveness Scale, and were prepared to sacrifice their own needs in order to achieve and maintain harmonious relationships (measured by the Need for Harmony Scale). Servaes et al (1999) compared 48 women with breast cancer with 49 healthy women with regard to alexithymia (inability to express emotion), emotional expression, assertiveness, repression, and distress. No difference was found between the two groups in alexithymia, expression of emotions, or willingness to talk with others about emotions generally. However, the patient group was more ambivalent about emotional expression and showed more restraint. Those authors report that the image of the breast cancer patient that emerged in the study was that of a person who has conflicting feelings with regard to expressing emotions, who is reserved, anxious, and self-effacing, and who represses aggression and impulsiveness. They conclude that emotional inhibition is a reaction to the disease rather than a personality trait. This conflicts with the findings of other studies, which suggests that this inhibition may be more of a state than a trait feature, and that suppression of emotions may be of aetiological significance in cancer, and may also be related to disease outcome (Temoshok, 1985). Whatever the underlying cause of emotional suppression, it does appear to be associated with poorer adjustment to cancer. Stanton et al (2000a) studied 92 women with breast cancer immediately after medical treatment and then 3 months later. Those who coped by expressing emotions had less distress and better physical health and vigour over the next 3 months. One possibility is that expressive coping acts as a vehicle for energizing active coping and fighting spirit.

The value of emotional expression

It is too simplistic to assert that the expression of emotions is therapeutic in its own right. Although catharsis is often described as one of the basic ingredients of psychotherapy (Frank, 1971), research findings in this area are not conclusive. Ventilation of feelings or catharsis only seems to be effective if it is accompanied by cognitive processing (Lewis and Bucher, 1992). Greenberg and Safran (1987) consider that the creation of new meaning when feelings are authentically experienced, owned, and expressed is a vital component of therapeutic change. They also view emotions as acting to facilitate problem solving by directing the individual towards constructive action. This link between emotional engagement and adaptive coping behaviour is present in the concept of emotional approach coping (Stanton et al, 2000b). The latter implies the active confrontation of thoughts and feelings about cancer. It is not surprising that this correlates positively with hope (Stanton et al 2000a), a construct described by Stanton as reflecting 'a sense of goal-directed determination, and ability to generate plans to achieve goals.' It has two components, namely emotional processing and emotional expression. In a recent study, Low et al (2010) found that emotional processing was associated with an increase in depressive symptoms and cancer-specific intrusive and avoidant thoughts at a later point in time, particularly for women with low levels of emotional support or self-efficacy. Emotional expression moderated the effect of cancer-specific intrusive thoughts on depressive symptoms at follow-up, and protected women with low levels of social support or emotional self-efficacy from increased distress. The acknowledgement and expression of feelings is integrally linked with construing the situation in a new way, and with developing appropriate plans for coping with the stress. Cognitive change is most effective if it takes place in the presence of affective arousal.

It is our clinical impression that giving patients the opportunity to tell their story is often one of the most important aspects of therapy. People who are going through the process of adjustment to their diagnosis or who are coming to terms with a new development, such as a recurrence, benefit from having time just to express their feelings. Social factors may have operated to prevent them from talking through their thoughts and feelings about cancer. Patients who are socially isolated have no one to talk to, patients who are experiencing relationship problems do not feel supported enough to express themselves, and, as we suggested earlier, many patients who are in good relationships do not want to burden their family. Studies have shown that a high proportion of patients with cancer, 86% in one study (Mitchell and Glicksman, 1977) wish that they could discuss their situation more fully with another person.

Processing or problem solving?

Although many patients benefit from ventilation of feelings, there are others who have spent a considerable time doing just that, but with little or no benefit. Indeed, the cognitive model predicts that talking about negative feelings will make one feel worse unless there is some reconstrual of the situation. Cancer patients who are depressed or anxious are often stuck in patterns of repetitive negative thoughts which they cannot re-evaluate. The challenge when working with this group of patients is to find the right balance between 'doing to' and 'being with' the person, between focusing on acceptance or focusing on change, and between facilitating emotional processing and encouraging active problem solving. As a general rule, when affect is overmodulated, emotional engagement and expression are required, but when affect is under-modulated, cognitive and behavioural techniques are needed. Wiser and Arnow (2001) have proposed some guidelines on when emotional expression should be facilitated in psychotherapy and when it should not. Moorey (1996) has suggested some factors to consider when deciding whether or not to encourage ventilation in individuals who are facing adverse life circumstances. The primary consideration is whether the person is going through a process of adjustment or is caught in a persistent negative mood state. If there is evidence for a continuing or arrested adjustment reaction, emotive techniques may be appropriate. However, if the person is markedly anxious or depressed, or if they might have difficulty in tolerating high levels of emotional arousal, more problem-oriented techniques are indicated.

Indications for facilitating emotional expression

These include the following:

1. recent onset of emotional distress in the setting of a specific change in cancer status (e.g. diagnosis, recurrence, clinic check-up)
2. markedly fluctuating emotional reactions
3. the presence of primary emotions (sadness rather than depression, fear rather than anxiety)
4. the absence of cognitive distortions (thought content is negative but appropriate)
5. significant beliefs about the negative impact of expressing emotions.

Indications for problem-focused interventions

These include the following:

1. prolonged negative mood state (anxiety, depression, anger)
2. affect overwhelming for patient
3. significant behavioural deficits (e.g. prolonged periods in bed because of depressed mood) or behavioural avoidance (e.g. chemotherapy phobia)
4. presence of maladaptive emotions and cognitive distortions (e.g. guilt, self-blame, pervasive hopelessness).

Facilitating emotional expression

In practice the distinction between ventilation and problem solving is not always so clear cut. It is always necessary to help the person to engage with their feelings and express them before using cognitive or behavioural interventions.

Without this, it is impossible to understand the personal meaning of the situation for the patient. The therapist always acknowledges the fact that any negative feeling is real for the patient, no matter how unrealistic it may be. This validation is important for establishing and maintaining the therapeutic alliance. The feeling must be acknowledged before moving on to the cognitive content of the problem. There is some empirical evidence that a good therapeutic alliance combined with emotional involvement (experiencing) on the part of the patient is associated with a better outcome in CBT for depression (Castonguay et al, 1996). There is also evidence that some therapist interventions are more likely to help patients to maintain a high level of emotional experiencing in CBT (Wiser and Goldfried, 1998).

There are a number of ways to encourage the experiencing of appropriate affect (for a more detailed discussion, see Greenberger and Safran, 1987):

1. Educate the patient about emotional reactions to cancer (normalization).
2. Be less active. Simply being silent for a while may allow feelings to emerge.
3. Use open-ended rather than closed questions.
4. Use reflective comments (e.g. 'I can understand how you feel').
5. Attend to emotionally relevant experience, and help the patient to attend to this too (e.g. 'What is that like for you now?' or 'How do you feel?').
6. Pay attention to the patient's manner of expression, facial and postural expressions, sighs, etc.
7. Keep the focus on experiencing in the here and now.
8. Use the 'poignancy criterion.' If the material feels poignant for the therapist, it is probably relevant to appropriate emotional expression.
9. When the patient moves to third-person language bring them back to the first person (e.g. 'You feel …').
10. Challenge negative thoughts and beliefs about emotional expression (Moorey, 1996).

Accepting emotions

Getting the patient to accept negative emotions can often break the circle of distress that they are experiencing. Teasdale (1983) described how people can get 'depressed about depression', by focusing on symptoms such as tiredness, lack of concentration, or lack of pleasurable activities. Clinical experience suggests that this also applies to people with cancer, and is not just restricted to depression. Patients frequently report that they feel guilty about their increased irritability and angry outbursts. If they can accept their anger, this may defuse the situation considerably. Accepting their emotions can also allow patients to step back and observe themselves more objectively. Various methods can be used by the patient, including the following:

1. counting to 10 or taking a deep breath before acting on the feeling, or trying to avoid it
2. saying 'This is a normal feeling – there is nothing wrong with feeling angry/ frightened/sad'
3. imagining that the emotion is like a wave, and that the patient is a surfer who rides the wave until it has gone.

Mindfulness

Mindfulness is a particular way of relating to emotions by accepting them without becoming completely immersed in them. It has been defined as 'the awareness that emerges through paying attention on purpose, in the present moment, and non-judgementally, to the unfolding of experience moment by moment' (Kabat-Zinn, 2003, p. 145). Cultivating mindfulness allows us to be fully aware of what is going on without being caught up in the experience to the extent that we lose ourselves. The overwhelming feelings that are generated by receiving bad news about cancer can seem as if they will go on for ever, and we can lose ourselves in thoughts like 'This will never stop. What am I going to do? I can't cope.' We quickly start to tell ourselves stories about how things are going to look, about what this means about us, and about what this will mean for our family, that take us away from our immediate present into worries about a future that is not here and may never arrive. The skill of mindfulness helps us to be present for whatever is happening as it happens, opening ourselves to the 'full catastrophe' (Kabat-Zinn, 1990) without disappearing into loops of worry. Ultimately this means being open to emotional experience without practising our usual ways of escaping through subtle or not so subtle avoidance.

Because it is counterintuitive to lean into our distress rather than away from it, mindfulness is usually taught as part of a programme (Kabat-Zinn, 1990) rather than as a technique. Mindfulness-based stress reduction is usually a 6- to 8-week group course, and has been used in people with cancer (Speca, 1999; Lengacher et al, 2009) (for a manual of mindfulness-based cognitive therapy for people with cancer, see Bartley, 2011).

However, mindfulness is still a natural skill which we all possess, and there are ways in which it can be incorporated into a course of APT to aid the acceptance of emotions, and to manage worry and ruminations. We shall suggest two mindfulness practices that patients might find helpful.

The 'breathing space' (Segal et al, 2002)

Whenever we gather our thoughts or notice that we have been daydreaming we are practising mindfulness. Learning to create a space in which to be present can be very helpful when we are caught up in the maelstrom of emotional reactions to life-threatening illness. The instructions for creating the breathing space are as follows:

1. Take the opportunity to step out of whatever you are doing and check in with what you are experiencing. Take note of what you can hear, what you are thinking, what emotions you are feeling, and what is happening in your body. Give yourself permission to just be with whatever is happening right now.

2. Now bring your attention down to your breath. Follow the in-breath and the out-breath, focusing on your nostrils, chest or belly, wherever feels most appropriate. Allow the breath to come naturally without trying to control it.

3. Now expand around your breath to pay attention to your whole body, noticing feelings of tension or lightness, following the changes in sensations as they occur moment by moment. Be kind to yourself and accept whatever you are feeling or sensing.

4. With this open awareness, come back to your situation ready to make decisions about how you can respond wisely rather than react blindly.

Mindfulness in everyday life

Practising mindfulness in everyday activities can create space to be more awake to what you are experiencing, and can also help to move you from worry and ruminations into 'here-and-now' experience. Patients are encouraged to take time to really pay attention to what they are doing —eating a meal and noticing the smells and flavours, fully experiencing the warmth and wetness of a shower, noticing the wind on their face and the feelings in their muscles as they take a walk. This can help them to take themselves out of automatic pilot mode, and with practice they can create 'worry-free zones' (Colette Hirsch, personal communication) where they can be mindful.

The therapist can explain the concept and practise the breathing space or mindful attention in the session, and then suggest that the patient tries them as homework. Useful information and instructions on how to practise mindfulness have been provided by Segal et al (2002) and Bartley (2011). Caution needs to be exercised if the patient is prone to dissociation, as these techniques may very occasionally trigger this.

Identifying and working with emotional cues

The following example, taken from a first session of APT, demonstrates how the therapist can identify possible areas of emotional significance from the cues that the patient presents. In this case the patient was a 55-year-old woman who had carcinoma of the cervix. As part of the assessment the therapist had asked about her family.

Patient: I've got no family of my own.

Therapist: Why is that? Have your parents died?

Patient: Yes. There's just my brother. I don't see anything of him and that's that.

(Here the therapist sensed that the patient was resentful of her brother not visiting. This statement, together with the first one, 'I've got no family of my own', suggested that the patient felt alone and deserted.)

Therapist: How long ago did your parents die?

Patient: My dad died five years ago, and my mum's been gone 13 years now.

Therapist: (The therapist senses from the patient's non-verbal reaction, which made her appear tense and sad, that this was still a significant loss). Were you very close to them?

Patient: Yeah (looking tearful).

Therapist: And you still miss them (emphatically stating the patient's feeling of loss).

Patient: (Nods, sobbing.)

Therapist: Just talking about it makes you feel upset.

Patient: That is one problem I never sorted out. That is the problem – you've hit it on the head.

Therapist: Who do you miss most?

Patient: My mother (sobbing).

Therapist: Your mother (repeating the patient's own words).

Patient: I nursed her till she died. … I did everything for her and it was her that I miss terribly. I never got over her death.

Having elicited this strong emotional reaction, the therapist was able to explore the meaning of this loss and to make some hypotheses about why it was still so vivid. Two significant factors seemed to emerge. First, the mother had been very close, and despite a long illness with cirrhosis of the liver she provided strong emotional support for the patient. In the second session the therapist asked the patient how her mother might have helped her to cope. The patient replied 'She would have worried about it for me. She would have told me it was going to be all right.' Her mother had shouldered all of her burdens and reassured her.

The therapist needed to construct a plan of action that both helped the woman to learn some coping strategies for herself, and also utilized her social support network. The second factor was the resonance that the patient's illness had set up with memories of her mother's death. Expressing her feelings about this, particularly admitting her own fears of a long lingering death, gave her a sense of relief.

Sometimes catharsis occurs later in therapy, in relation to a key issue. Jenny was helped by being allowed to express some of her fears about her child. Halfway through treatment she visited a colleague in hospital. This woman also had cancer and was dying. Jenny handled the situation extremely well at the time, but later experienced a delayed reaction to it and became quite upset. When we explored this during the therapy session, she spoke of her feelings of identification with her friend, and her fears of death. The therapist encouraged her to express her negative feelings openly, and she cried for the first time in treatment. Her main fears undoubtedly concerned her son and his future. She described feeling guilty 'for doing such a terrible thing to him.' She also worried about his future development if she died. The therapist used empathy and reflection to allow her both to talk about this and to experience the emotions associated with it. This in itself was helpful, as she had probably been thinking about it but was hesitant about facing up to it.

Later in the session the therapist helped Jenny to clarify her realistic sadness about the thought of leaving her son, and to distinguish this from the distorted thinking that was associated with her guilt. She quickly saw that she could not hold herself responsible for the cancer or for the effect of her death on her child, but that she could do everything in her power to make sure that his future was provided for. The session ended with a review of the objective factors relating to her disease, namely that she had early breast cancer which had been successfully treated, to help her to continue with her fight against the disease.

Working with denial

In a recent review of the literature on denial, Vos and de Haes (2007) reported that the prevalence of denial of the diagnosis among cancer patients was in the range 4–47%, while denial of the impact occurred in 8–70% of patients and denial of affect occurred in 18–42% of patients. Cultural background and age were associated with denial, but gender and type of cancer were not. Denial appears to decrease over time. The relationship between denial, other coping strategies, and adjustment is still not clear from research evidence, but clinically we would not automatically challenge denial, as it may be the most adaptive way for the patient to cope with the current situation. If there are objective signs that the distorted positive thinking is harming the patient, it should be tackled using the techniques for encouraging emotional expression described above, and the techniques of reality testing that are described in Chapter 9. Situations in which it might be necessary to challenge denial include the following:

1. when denial of the existence or seriousness of cancer prevents the patient from engaging with treatment

2. when denial on the part of the patient or their partner causes such a mismatch in their perception of the disease that communication problems and emotional distress occur

3. when denial is not an effective coping strategy, and breakthrough anxiety or depression occurs

4. when denial prevents active problem solving (e.g. a dying man does not make the necessary plans for the future of his family).

Encouraging and channelling expression of anger

As with denial, anger can be addressed through emotion-based and cognitive behavioural techniques. Some of the techniques for challenging angry thoughts are described in Chapter 10. Here we shall present some ways to encourage the expression of appropriate anger and to channel it constructively.

Ventilation

When a patient perceives their situation as unjust, their emotional reaction will tend to be one of anger. Most people will find some way of expressing this openly, or will at least accept the emotion. Those who suppress anger feel that it is unsafe, or even morally wrong, to get angry. Cognitive avoidance may also come into play to prevent the person from attending to the thoughts associated with this negative affect, so there may be denial of the anger. However, the cognitive processes associated with the perceived insult will continue to operate. A self-destructive smouldering resentment may then be set up.

In many situations, merely expressing the anger may be therapeutic in its own right. Ventilation may be easier than trying to challenge the irrational basis of the anger, as this implicitly reinforces the injunction against angry feelings. Simply telling someone that you are angry with him can prevent the resentment from escalating. For those who bottle up their feelings it may be helpful to set aside times when they can be 'emotional.' Once ventilation has produced some emotional relief, it is then possible to examine the cognition associated with the emotion and find alternative ways of dealing with it in the future.

Positive action

It is not always possible to express anger openly. If anger is felt towards God or the boss, this cannot be expressed face to face. Activities that allow the person to let off steam (e.g. going jogging, punching a pillow, etc.) can be planned. An alternative to letting off steam is to adopt a problem-solving approach. The energy from the anger can then be channelled or 'sublimated' into action that overcomes the perceived problem. For instance, if the patient says 'The doctor didn't give me enough chance to ask questions', there are a number of actions that the patient can take to achieve the goal of finding out certain things he or she wants to know. The doctor can be confronted directly, or alternatively other sources of information can be consulted. It may be necessary to teach the patient assertiveness skills to enable them to achieve the goal of the positive action. Unassertive people may quickly switch from anger to helplessness in the way that they construe a situation. Getting them to do something to overcome the obstacle is a means of increasing their self-efficacy. More behavioural and cognitive techniques for dealing with anger are described in Chapter 10.

Summary

As well as the emphasis on cognitions and behaviour, APT attaches great importance to emotions. Emotions, cognitions, and behaviour are integrally connected in the adjustment process. Negative emotions need to be experienced and expressed in order to cognitively and emotionally process the trauma of a life-threatening illness. We have presented some guidelines on when emotional processing should be encouraged and when it is more appropriate to pursue a problem-solving focus. Techniques for facilitating emotional expression and for working with denial and anger have been described. In the next two chapters we shall address the behavioural and cognitive components of this cognitive–behavioural–affective system.

Chapter 8

Behavioural techniques

The primary aim of the behavioural interventions in APT is to enable the patient to make maximum use of the activities available within the constraints of the disease. This helps to foster a fighting spirit and a sense of personal control. Behavioural techniques can also be used to cope with stress (relaxation training), and as a means of changing attitudes (behavioural experiments). Since this is a *cognitive* behavioural therapy, behaviour change is usually designed to test specific thoughts or beliefs. Ideally these interventions should come from the conceptualization of the patient's problems. For instance, the meaning of cancer for one woman was that she was now alone and isolated. The therapist helped her to test this belief by asking her to contact friends and assess their reactions to her invitation to meet. She found that although some of them said they were busy, or sounded uncomfortable talking to her because of her illness, most were very pleased to hear from her and eager to help in any way that they could. In other cases, behavioural techniques may be directed at alleviating anxiety or depression. The rationale for any intervention should always be explained to the patient, and incorporated within the shared conceptualization. Behavioural tasks are collaboratively developed as homework assignments. They may be suggested as methods to distract the patient from negative thoughts, to test unhelpful beliefs, or to build feelings of self-efficacy. It is important to establish that the patient understands the rationale for any assignment in order to increase the likelihood of the assignment being carried out.

In this chapter we shall describe the following behavioural techniques:

- relaxation training
- activity scheduling
- graded task assignment
- planning for the future
- behavioural experiments.

Illustrations will be given of how to work behaviourally with threats to survival in anxiously preoccupied and hopeless patients, and how to deal with anxiety and depression that arise from threats to self-image and self-esteem.

Relaxation training

Anxiety is one of the commonest symptoms among people with cancer. In the cognitive model this emotion results from the recognition of a significant threat to survival or to the view of the self and the world, combined with a reduction in confidence that there are resources available to cope with the threat. As the disease is genuinely life-threatening and no one can be certain that their own resources or the treatment they receive will guarantee cure, anxiety is a realistic and natural reaction. What might be termed 'normal' anxiety merges imperceptibly into pathological anxiety. The extent to which anxiety symptoms are a focus in therapy is determined by their severity in relation to the objective threats of cancer, their duration and interference with everyday life, and whether or not the patient regards them as a problem.

Relaxation does not have to be confined to regular sessions at home. It can be used as a coping strategy in stressful situations. Patients can be taught to relax whenever they feel tense or anxious. Breathing exercises may be more helpful than muscle relaxation, as they can be done when the patient is sitting or walking. The therapist must analyse the anxiety-provoking situation closely and find cues that can act as reminders of when to relax. The patient practises relaxing on cue during the session. These exercises can then be combined with distraction, self-instruction, and cognitive restructuring to produce an anxiety management package that is tailored for each patient. Situations in which this might be used include waiting for and undergoing radiotherapy or chemotherapy, and going into new social situations.

Relaxation training is a simple and effective method for giving people rapid control of their anxiety symptoms. Two forms of relaxation are taught, namely progressive muscle relaxation and breathing exercises. Research suggests that these are equally effective, but individual patients may prefer one or the other. People who have pulmonary problems or suffer from shortness of breath may not find breathing the best focus for relaxation training. Imagery techniques can provide a useful method for these patients.

The exercises described below are instructions to patients from the handbook developed by the Beth Israel Hospital (Borysenko et al, 1986). These can be used as a guide for teaching patients the two types of relaxation.

Progressive muscle relaxation

Each of the following tension/relaxation exercises is done in conjunction with the breathing exercises. Tense each body part to its maximum as you breathe in. Hold it for as long as is comfortable. Then let go of the tension gradually as you exhale.

1. Make fists with your toes. Relax.

2. Pull your feet back, bringing your toes towards your knees. Relax.

3. Tense the muscles of your thighs as if you were trying to lift your legs against a weight. Relax.

4. Pinch your buttocks in and up, making them hard, as if you were seated upon a rock. Relax.

5. Take a large chest breath and pull your abdomen in, hardening it. Relax.

6. Take a large chest breath and tense your whole upper body. Relax.

7. Make fists with your hands. Relax.

8. Pull your hands back at the wrists, as if to bend the hand up towards the elbow. Relax.

9. Raise your shoulders up to your ears. Relax.

10. Raise your eyebrows and furrow your forehead. Relax.

11. Squeeze your eyes shut. Relax.

12. Smile, pulling back the corners of your mouth and baring your teeth. Relax.

Breathing exercises

1. *Awareness of breathing*: as you continue your activities, become aware of your breathing. Inhale deeply, exhale completely, and focus attention on belly breathing. This exercise can be as short as one breath or as long as several minutes.

2. *10 to 1 countdown*: close your eyes. Take a deep breath and exhale completely. Begin to breathe diaphragmatically. On the next out-breath repeat the number 10. As you exhale, feel the tension drain out in a wave from your head, all the way down your body, and out of the soles of your feet. On each subsequent out-breath, count back one number until you reach 1, continuing to use the out-breath as an opportunity to release muscle tension.

3. *Letting go of tension with the out-breath*: muscle tension naturally diminishes on the out-breath as the body lets go to the pull of gravity. Just as in the 10 to 1 countdown, any breath can be used as an opportunity to let go of tension (from Borysenko et al, 1986).

The usual procedure is to teach the patient relaxation during the session and to ask them to continue this regularly as homework. The exact instructions will vary, but the therapist normally suggests that the patient should practise once or twice a day for 20 minutes at a time. Patients who have sleeping difficulties can try relaxation in bed.

When teaching this technique it is necessary to obtain feedback from the patient about how they are feeling and what they are doing. Summarizing the steps in relaxation before and after teaching the procedure is helpful, and the instructions can be reinforced by giving the patient a handout and/or an audiotape. If the session is taped, the patient will be able to take away a cassette and use this at home. Alternatively, a commercial relaxation tape may be used. Neil Fiore (1984) has produced a relaxation tape specifically for people with cancer. If the patient's partner is present, they can be included in the relaxation exercise.

Once the relaxation response has been learned, the person can practise using it in more stressful situations. They can begin by leaving cues around the house to remind them to relax (e.g. Post-it notes on mirrors, the television, etc.), and practise counting back from 5 or 10, allowing themselves to become more relaxed at each step. Once they have practised, they will find that they can focus on 'lowering their emotional temperature' by counting backwards and concentrating on relaxing.

Activity scheduling

Cancer can be a demoralizing experience that leads to a progressive reduction in activities. Sometimes this starts when fatigue, nausea, or other symptoms are induced by treatment. While most people are able to return to a normal life when their course of radiotherapy or chemotherapy has ended, some remain stuck in a state of inactivity. Symptoms of anxiety can cause avoidance of social situations. Depression causes social withdrawal, loss of motivation, and loss of interest in pleasant activities. A young married woman with local recurrence of breast cancer wanted to leave her job and buy a new house. She and her husband kept saying to themselves that they would wait until she was cured before they made any plans for the future. As a result, any possible changes in their lives were met with the response 'We'll wait and see.' Not only major plans but also short-term goals like decorating the house were put off, and the patient felt a sense of dejection and frustration.

One way of overcoming this inertia is to encourage rewarding activities. For this couple, planning to decorate a room together demonstrated that it was still possible to get on with ordinary life even with the threat of cancer unresolved. Behavioural interventions can foster a fighting spirit and also give the person strategies for positive avoidance. Positive avoidance is the active, conscious behavioural and cognitive avoidance that allows the patient to concentrate on everyday life without constantly thinking about cancer. The capacity to put cancer out of one's thoughts for at least some of the time seems to be a characteristic of many people who are coping well with their illness. Positive avoidance can become a flexible, conscious strategy that gives the patient control over how much time they spend on cancer-related thoughts as opposed to other areas of life.

Functions of activity scheduling

Information gathering

The therapist finds out when the patient feels low and how this is related to their behaviour. For instance, a depressed man might feel most depressed in the evenings when he is watching TV. The negative thoughts associated with this can be identified and activities scheduled which are less passive, such as visiting friends. Patients rate activities for pleasure (P 0–10) and mastery (M 0–10), which allows the therapist to identify which activities have the most antidepressant effect (see below).

Distraction

By scheduling activities for times when the patient is most preoccupied by anxious or depressive thoughts, he or she can be distracted from those thoughts. At times when negative thoughts are very strong, it can be difficult to counter them. Distraction may be the most effective coping strategy to use until the person's mood improves. The patient, the therapist and the patient's partner work together to identify the most effective distracting activities, which are then to be used at times during the day when the patient is most vulnerable.

Increasing self-efficacy

Behaviours that give the patient a feeling of control or mastery can be particularly helpful in combating feelings of hopelessness and helplessness. Increasing a sense of mastery may also improve symptoms. Byma et al (2009) found that during an 8-week nurse intervention for symptom management, mastery (defined as the personal control felt by the patient over occurrences perceived to have an important effect on their life) was a predictor of pain reduction but, interestingly, did not predict a reduction in fatigue. The partner can be a useful informant who knows what gave the patient feelings of success or control.

Increasing motivation

Many people believe that motivation is derived from inspiration. However, according to the cognitive behavioural model, motivation results from seeing the positive effects of behaviour. The more rewarding an activity is, the more likely we are to engage in it again. The demoralized patient sees no point in doing anything, and falls into a self-defeating cycle of inactivity and loss of motivation.

Challenging negative attitudes

Patients who are finding it difficult to cope assume that cancer now rules their life and they no longer have any control. Engaging in activities that used to be important to the patient demonstrates to them that life can return to normal. As always, behavioural change can act as a powerful means of achieving cognitive change, by disproving negative beliefs.

Using activity scheduling

Behavioural assignments are a potent component of CBT. They can be used as single activities (e.g. setting the task of writing to an old friend whom the patient had lost touch with), or they can be used within the framework of an *activity schedule*. This can provide a structure for the day or the week. If a patient is too ill to work, the week can suddenly look very empty without the familiar framework that was provided by their job. Scheduling in something to do each day, however small, can introduce structure to the week and give the person events which they can look forward to. A weekly activity schedule is often given to the patient at the end of the first session. A copy of a blank schedule can be found in Appendix 3. This is introduced with the rationale which is tailored to the patient's particular problems. Two examples are given below.

Anxious preoccupation

'Cancer is such a frightening condition that it takes up much of a person's time in thinking about treatment and what the future holds. Sometimes this means that the rest of life just gets squeezed out. Are there things that you are avoiding or no longer doing because of your worries?'

Helplessness/hopelessness

'You have told me how bleak your future looks to you, and you say that you can't see the point in doing anything. We find that many people get stuck in a vicious circle. They give up things because they see no point in them, and then they get few rewards from life, so they become even more depressed and unmotivated. If you would like to try, I think we can break this vicious circle.'

As a general principle, when using activity scheduling it is best to find out when certain activities give patients a sense of control or achievement (*mastery*) and *pleasure*. They may find this difficult at first, especially if they are depressed and are not deriving any pleasure from life. Sometimes asking about past behaviours which the patient might have given up, or about activities that they have always wanted to take up, can generate a useful list. The partner can act as a co-therapist here by reminding the patient about activities which he or she used to find rewarding. The patient's strengths should be used as a guide for planning new activities, and again the partner can be involved in this exercise.

Some examples of mastery and pleasure experiences are listed below:

Mastery experiences

1. Driving a car for the first time since the patient's operation.
2. Taking up a new hobby.
3. Becoming a hospital visitor.
4. Looking after their grandchildren for the afternoon.
5. Writing thank-you letters to friends who have sent get well cards.

Pleasure experiences

1. Going to the cinema.
2. Reading a book.
3. Going on holiday.
4. Buying new clothes.
5. Going out for dinner.

The tasks need to be tailored to the individual's personality. Some people find doing things for others rewarding, while others find personal success more satisfying. When constructing the activity schedule, patients grade their experience with regard to mastery and pleasure from 0 to 10. Activities that are rated high on mastery (M) or pleasure (P) can be scheduled more frequently in the next week. Constructing a timetable of the week often reveals blank spaces when the person is vulnerable to negative thoughts and feelings. For instance, an anxious woman found from her record of activities that when her husband was doing night work she would spend a lot of the evening worrying about her cancer. The therapist suggested that she should decide what strategies she might use when this next happened (e.g. having a book or writing paper by her bed, making a decision to get up and make a cup of tea when she woke up).

Cognitive distortions can contribute to behavioural deficits. All-or-nothing thinking occurs particularly frequently. Fatigue and depression prevent people from doing things as well as they used to, and many patients will then start to think that either they must do things as well as before or they won't do them at all. Rating mastery and pleasure can help the patient to start grading these experiences, rather than seeing them in black-and-white terms. Another common distortion is minimization (e.g. 'That doesn't count – I was able to do it every day before'). After a course of chemotherapy, just making a meal may be a major achievement. Looking at what the patient is doing provides a means of identifying and challenging such negative thinking.

For some patients, behavioural techniques may be the most helpful component of treatment. There is evidence that behavioural activation alone can be a highly effective treatment for depression in people with cancer (Hopko et al, 2005).

Graded task assignments

The ability to do things as fast and efficiently as before the onset of cancer can be impaired for several reasons. In early disease, physical causes (e.g. the side-effects of treatment) or psychological factors (e.g. depression) can affect the performance of tasks that the patient previously found easy. In later disease the effects of pain or fatigue can be debilitating. It can be difficult to adjust to this. The result is often that the patient either strives to do everything at the same pace as before the illness, or gives up altogether. We shall describe cognitive techniques for dealing with this all-or-nothing thinking in the next chapter. The behavioural concomitant of these is *graded task assignment*. People who are depressed or physically ill cannot be expected to return immediately to their previous levels of activity. Tasks can be divided into their individual components and completed one step at a time. For example, the husband of a depressed patient worked out a plan for gradually increasing joint social activities after his wife returned home from hospital. Starting with trips to the shops, they moved on to increasingly difficult tasks. Patients recovering from an operation might set themselves the task of gradually increasing their level of physical exercise on a daily basis, starting with walking around their flat, then moving on to walking in the garden, walking round the block, and so on. By breaking down large tasks into small steps, each step forward becomes an achievement that can be celebrated, motivating the person to move on to the next one.

Planning for the future

The temporal focus of the patient's daily life can be important in therapy, as the helpless/hopeless patient tends to view the future in an overly pessimistic way.

Some patients have very high standards and expect to be able to perform at the same level every day. This is not possible if they are receiving unpleasant treatments that cause fatigue or nausea. However, encouraging the patient to titrate their activity level to their physical strength can overcome this problem. The focus of attention can change to 'one day at a time', and graded tasks can be used to increase activities in a stepwise fashion.

Many patients adopt the opposite attitude to the future. They say 'I'm just taking one day at a time', and limit their lives as a result. For these individuals, planning ahead is the best strategy. For patients who are convinced that they will be dead within a month, but really have a life expectancy of years, a 'lifetime goals exercise' may prove a dramatic challenge to their hopelessness (Lakein, 1973). Here the therapist asks the patient to think about what their goals would be if they knew that they could live a normal lifespan. The aim of this exercise is to extend the patient's timescale and open up ideas about the future. This can then be repeated with the instructions that the patient now knows that they can live an active life for a year, so what would be their goals? The final step is to ask the patient to decide what they could do in the *next week* to start the process of moving towards these goals. Thus, whatever the real prognosis, the patient can now say that significant steps are being taken towards achieving important aims.

The time span for planning rewarding activities is best decided by the patient and their partner. Objective knowledge about the disease needs to be taken into account. Some patients can afford to plan years ahead, while others might be better off thinking in terms of weeks or months. A statement of intent to go on holiday in a year's time is a powerful stand against the disease.

Behavioural experiments

Many of the interventions in CBT are set up as experiments to test the individual's beliefs about him- or herself, the world, or the future. A behavioural test can prove far more effective in changing negative attitudes than several sessions of discussion. The activity scheduling and task assignments described above can be presented to the patient as experiments, as neither the therapist nor the patient know the outcome for certain beforehand. By examining the thought and its meaning, it is possible to devise a specific prediction about what would happen if the patient tests their negative belief. Behavioural experiments consist of the following five steps:

1. Elicit the thought or belief.
2. Make a prediction of what would happen if this belief was correct/incorrect (this should be as specific and operational as possible).

3. Devise an experiment to test this prediction.

4. Carry out the experiment.

5. Evaluate the outcome.

Example 1

Thought: I can't concentrate on anything.

Prediction: I won't be able to find anything I can concentrate on for more than 5 minutes.

Experiment: 1. Find something that I can concentrate on for 5 minutes.
2. Increase the time I spend on it by 1 minute each day.

Outcome: 1. I concentrated on reading the paper for 5 minutes, and then got so interested that I found I had been reading for 15 minutes.
2. I was able to increase the time reading by 5 minutes each day.

My concentration isn't as bad as I thought.

Example 2

Thought: Because of my mastectomy my husband doesn't want me sexually.

Prediction: Men will not be interested in women if they don't have attractive breasts.

Experiment: 1. Find out from husband what attracts him to women (e.g. personality, dress, physical appearance).
2. How many of these attributes do you have?

Outcome: My husband values personality and a sense of humour most in a partner. He says he loves and wants me just as much as before. Perhaps he isn't as put off by me as I thought.

Experiments can be set as homework, or they can be undertaken during the session. In both of the above examples the experiment could have been done with the therapist present. The first patient could be asked to read something for 5 minutes and report on how easy it was to concentrate. In the second case, the therapist might ask the partner to list all of the things he finds attractive about women, with the patient present.

Behavioural experiments during the session are of great value when working with patients' anxiety. If a patient is suffering from panic attacks, the catastrophic belief about the physical symptoms of anxiety needs to be elicited, and this can then be tested in the session. Feelings of breathlessness can be misinterpreted as signs that the patient is going to be unable to breathe and will suffocate. The therapist can get the patient to induce panic feelings by asking him or her to voluntarily hyperventilate in the session.

Example 3

Thought: When I get breathless it means I'm going to suffocate.

Prediction: 1. If this is really a physical problem, I won't be able to bring it on by simply overbreathing.

               2. If I don't control my breathing I'll suffocate.

Experiment: Hyperventilate together with the therapist in the session. Don't try to control your breathing.

Outcome: 1. The breathing exercise brought on the same symptoms as those I have during a panic attack.

               2. When I didn't try to control my breathing the breathlessness went away more quickly.

               This is probably anxiety, not a problem with my breathing. If I let myself breathe more freely, I'll actually feel better, not worse.

Sometimes behavioural experiments do not have the desired result. A depressed patient comes back and reports that the homework was a disaster. She phoned her friends as agreed and they were all too busy to see her. The meaning of this for the patient can be examined. What was her interpretation of their responses? Could they really be busy after all? Is she selectively attending to the negative parts of their replies? It may transpire that one of her friends said she was booked up this week but would love to see the patient another time, but the patient had deleted this from her conclusion. A 'failed' experiment will always provide information about the patient's thoughts and how they may have inadvertently behaved in a way that prevented the task from succeeding. If a genuinely negative response to an experiment like this is received, cognitive work can be done to decatastrophize the meaning of rejection.

Using behavioural techniques with the anxiously preoccupied patient

The patient with anxious preoccupation views cancer as a major threat that he or she feels unable to control. The future seems horrifyingly uncertain. Uncertainty about the prognosis and doubts about whether one has the strength to cope are issues for all people with cancer, but for the anxious patient they assume overwhelming importance. Behavioural tasks can help both to increase control and to reduce uncertainty. The following case is an example of how a simple behavioural intervention can effect a change in attitude.

This use of activity scheduling helps to change the focus from cancer to other areas of the patient's life. For the anxiously preoccupied patient who is concerned about their inability to control the disease, this new approach can be introduced in the following way:

Mary was a 56-year-old widow who had been treated for cancer of the cervix in 1984. She received two courses of chemotherapy, followed by radical radio-therapy to the whole pelvis. She then underwent two caesium insertions. The tumour did not respond completely, and recurred 6 months after treatment. Mary responded well to a second course of treatment, but although she was free of recurrence, she could not free herself of the belief that the cancer was still there.

An analysis of her activities during the week clearly showed that she was spending a great deal of time alone, with very little contact with other people. The contact that she did have was limited to working in her sister's shop from time to time. Although she did this job well, she was in constant fear of criticism, frequently thinking to herself 'They don't want me here ... I'm always in the wrong.' Her thoughts about the illness were most marked when she was alone and feeling bored. These thoughts also became entangled with other automatic thoughts about not being needed. During the session she was able to talk honestly about how part of her believed the doctors when they told her she was free of disease, but when she was alone she was unable to cope with her fears.

The behavioural intervention was aimed at distracting Mary from her cancer-related thoughts when she was not able to deal with them. It was also framed to provide her with more control over areas of her life that she *could* influence. The therapist began by using the Weekly Activity Schedule, and asked her to plan an activity for each day. Activities were selected that gave her a sense of self-efficacy. She chose decorating her house as one goal which she had been putting off for a long time. Going for walks was another pleasant activity that she wished to pursue. Her self-confidence improved as she successfully painted a room in her house. The positive feedback from these behaviours also began to challenge her beliefs about still having cancer. She said 'If I was still ill, I wouldn't be able to do the things I've been doing in the last week.'

As the therapy progressed, Mary undertook more adventurous tasks. She began to get involved with a local charity (which gave her an area of her life where she could feel needed), and she also started to explore ways in which she could be more assertive. In this case, activity scheduling formed only part of the total APT programme.

Mary also attended a relaxation group which equipped her with self-help skills for dealing with anxiety. As she progressed through therapy she was taught to identify her self-defeating thoughts, and she eventually became able to challenge her beliefs that she was unwanted and a failure.

'When we see that there is little we can do to exert control in a particular area of our life, we feel helpless. This may extend unnecessarily to other areas, where we in fact do have a lot of control.'

The therapist then encourages the patient to look at the advantages and disadvantages of focusing exclusively on the disease. Patients with more advanced disease may find phrases such as 'You can't have control over your death, but you can control your life' useful for reorienting themselves.

Anxious patients often try in vain to cope with their cancer by desperately seeking more and more information, or trying one alternative cure after another. APT directs and channels their energies with more skilful and adaptive methods of coping. Sometimes it is necessary to put a ban on information seeking if it is just feeding into a cycle of anxious preoccupation. At other times it is best to help the patient to become a more effective information seeker (e.g. by rehearsing questions for the doctors, clarifying the reasons why particular information is needed, etc.).

Another way of promoting personal control is by helping the patient to adopt a realistic approach to staying healthy. Taking steps to improve the prognosis is not confined to the medical treatment of the disease. There are many things which the patient can do to promote their own health. These include taking regular exercise where possible, giving up smoking, eating a healthy diet, and finding ways of relaxing. These activities, which are healthy in their own right, may also contribute to the fight against the disease. The patient and their partner can make a list together of the things that they can do to exert some influence over the disease. This can become a brainstorming exercise, where the couple just note down anything that is even remotely possible, from vitamin C to aromatherapy. The act of writing ideas down on paper is another step in countering the belief that there is nothing the patient can do. The anxious patient may be using these strategies already, but therapy helps to put their usefulness in perspective. For instance, a woman with ovarian cancer was exhausting herself swimming 60 lengths a session and jogging every day. In her case it was necessary to discuss and plan appropriate and moderate use of healthy exercise.

Similar methods can be used to deal with uncertainty about the outcome. Behavioural techniques can be used to move the focus away from the prognosis of the disease. The therapist could say 'We cannot do much to reduce the risk of recurrence, but we can help you to reduce uncertainty elsewhere in your life.' Activities can be scheduled that are predictable and pleasurable. Engaging in interesting activities also helps to distract the patient from their preoccupation with recurrence. For example, a woman who had repeated concerns that the cancer had recurred in various parts of her body found that her anxiety lessened over Christmas. The pleasure of looking after her young children distracted her from focusing on her disease.

Using behavioural techniques with the helpless/hopeless patient

For the patient with a helpless/hopeless response to the disease there is no longer uncertainty and doubt, but a profound pessimism about the future. They are convinced that nothing can be done to control the disease. Activity scheduling may be even more helpful for these patients than for anxious patients.

Jenny was a 45-year-old teacher. Cancer of the breast (T2 N1b) was discovered by her general practitioner, and she underwent local excision of the tumour, followed by radiotherapy. After starting radiotherapy she felt depressed, hopeless, and angry. She was concerned about stiffness in her arm, and feared that she would not be able to carry on with her job if she was to receive chemotherapy. She was divorced and had an 8-year-old son. Neither of her parents were alive, and she had very little social support from relatives or friends.

The first target of therapy was a feeling of hopelessness. The therapist explored what goals Jenny might have for the future if she was cured of cancer. This initially proved difficult, partly because of her depressed mood and partly because she regarded any personal goals as selfish. She identified goals which included visiting a friend in France, moving house, doing some creative writing, getting fit, finding appropriate schooling for her son, and engaging in more joint activities with her son. She agreed to try out some of these activities as part of the programme to give her more experiences of success and pleasure, and to help to structure her time.

At the end of the session the therapist asked for feedback, and Jenny said 'What's the point in doing these things to cheer myself up if I will be dead soon anyway?' This automatic thought required a cognitive intervention in order to ensure that the homework assignment would be a success. The therapist helped Jenny to consider some of the advantages that might result from improving her mood, regardless of the prognosis for her disease. The rationale for activity scheduling was repeated, and the homework was framed as an experiment ('Let's see what happens if you try some of these things').

Over the next two weeks Jenny's hopelessness decreased and she felt less overwhelmed by her negative automatic thoughts. She carried out the tasks that she had set herself, and started to take some time for herself during the day. She also started a light exercise programme. Activity scheduling laid the groundwork for more specific cognitive and behavioural interventions over the course of therapy (see Table 8.1).

Focusing on the quality of life enhances personal control over the areas of a person's activities that are unrelated to cancer. By encouraging experiences that foster a sense of mastery and control, the therapist helps the patient to start to interact with the world in an active way again. The concept of mastery can be explained and the patient asked to make a list of activities which might promote it. Their partner can be involved in this exercise. Another approach is to set up an experiment in which the patient tries out some of these behaviours and rates them according to the degree of control that they feel they have when engaging in them. The activities must be tailored to the individual and, as with all procedures in CBT, are promoted in a collaborative way so that the patient understands the rationale for the experiment and takes an active part in its construction.

Activities that are associated with feelings of control can range from doing the laundry to making a model. The patient should be encouraged to set their sights realistically. A simple activity, such as making a cup of tea, when done during a course of chemotherapy may be much more difficult and complex than when the patient is well.

The partner can be included in this approach, ideally as much as possible. The relationship should be explored to see whether there any interpersonal factors that are contributing to the feeling of helplessness. Some partners start to do all of the work about the house and do not let the patient with cancer do anything. If this is the case, there needs to be negotiation of a contract whereby the ill partner can do as much as possible within the confines of the illness. The healthy partner has to learn to accept as well as to give. This may require specific tasks to be set, such as getting the patient to do things for their partner to thank them for what they are doing.

The helpless patient may report negative cognitions about the extent to which their health can be influenced by anyone else. Behavioural tasks can be designed to challenge these helpless attitudes. A fighting spirit can be fostered by showing the patient how they can actively contribute to their recovery.

Following medical advice

This simple strategy involves reframing the locus of control in the doctor–patient relationship. Although the patient may have little say with regard to the choice of particular treatments, they do have a choice over whether or not they comply with the treatment. Treatment compliance is not a passive phenomenon, but is in fact an active course which the patient has chosen. Keeping appointments, taking medication regularly, and attending for blood tests are

Table 8.1 Weekly activity schedule for a helpless/hopeless patient with breast cancer

Time	Monday	Tuesday	Wednesday	Thursday	Friday	Saturday	Sunday
9–10 a.m.	Travelled to hospital for treatment	Travelled to hospital for treatment	Travelled to hospital for treatment	Travelled to hospital for treatment	Travelled to hospital for treatment		
10–11 a.m.	Travelled home		Travelled home	Travelled home	Travelled home		Laundry
11 a.m. –12 noon	Laundry		Went to post office	Tea and chat with friends	Tea with friends	Shopping	
12–1 p.m.			Lunch		Lunch at friend's house	Listened to tape of therapy session	Travelled to meet sister
1–2 p.m.			Met a friend for a drink	Lunch and housework		Lunch	
2–3 p.m.	Gardening		Went for a walk	Visit from colleague at work	Shopping	Bought a book	Lunch with sister
3–4 p.m.	Collected son	45 minutes' writing	Visited next-door neighbour	Collected son from school	Collected son from school		Walk
4–5 p.m.	20 minutes' writing Took son to football lesson	Collected son Drove him to football	Collected son	Shopping			Visited friend and sister for tea
5–6 p.m.	Walked home	Football lesson				Cooking	
6–7 p.m.	Collected son	Supper	Supper	Supper			Travelled home
7–8 p.m.	Supper Put child to bed	Put child to bed	Put child to bed		Supper at friend's house	Supper	Washing up. etc.
8–12 p.m.	Watched news Exercises	Watched news Exercises	Watched news Exercises	News Phone calls Exercises	Home	Reading Exercises	Ironing Put son to bed

all ways in which the patient acts to increase their chances of recovery. Each outpatient appointment represents a conscious choice to work with the doctors in fighting the disease. This can be further emphasized by considering the consequences of not complying with treatment.

Information seeking

The helpless/hopeless person can be helped to take more control of the illness by being directed to appropriate sources of information (e.g. booklets explaining the illness, books written by patients, etc.). The patient can be encouraged to approach their doctor with questions about the disease. The medical consultation is a frightening situation where all the power resides in the doctor, so it may be necessary to work with the patient beforehand in order to maximize the likelihood that they will ask effective questions and obtain appropriate answers. Writing down questions so that they are not forgotten in the outpatients department is a simple procedure that may prove useful. Other patients may need to rehearse or role play with the therapist what they want to say to their doctor.

This technique also provides valuable information about the patient's automatic thoughts in the situation. In order to be an effective information seeker, the patient has to learn to be specific in their questioning. To ease the patient's task, the therapist can inform the doctor that the patient has been encouraged to ask specific questions about treatment. This technique can prove a powerful mastery experience. It also serves to increase confidence in the medical staff, which in turn increases the patient's belief in the doctor's control over the disease. This can be taken one step further by examining the patient's confidence in the doctor and the hospital. Where appropriate, cognitive techniques such as reality testing are used to establish the credentials of the therapeutic team with the patient. With a disease such as cancer, where a patient may not be able to contribute as much to their own health as with other illnesses, it is correspondingly important that there should be trust of and effective communication with those treating the patient.

The choice of strategy will depend on the individual patient's problems. As always the therapist needs to be aware of the delicate balance between confronting negative thoughts and feelings about cancer, and helping the patient to distract him- or herself from overwhelming negative thoughts.

Further applications of behavioural techniques

So far we have been considering the use of behavioural techniques to cope with the threat that cancer represents to survival. Concerns about the progression of the disease and life expectancy are often accompanied by concerns about the impact that cancer has on key areas of the person's life. In a study of patients with newly diagnosed cancer, Harrison et al (1994) found that 50% of patients reported the current illness as a *major or moderate concern*, and 22% were concerned about the future. Patients was also worried about the effects of treatment (24%), physical symptoms (18%), and inability to do things (18%). The distinction between threat to survival and threat to other aspects of the patient's life is often arbitrary in clinical practice. The patient with an anxious preoccupation whom we considered earlier had chronically low self-esteem. The hopeless patient had also had problems with interpersonal relationships in the past, and saw the side-effects of her treatment for cancer (a stiff arm following radiotherapy) as a sign that she was an invalid. Behavioural techniques can be used to address problems that arise within these other aspects of the patient's life (e.g. treatment, physical disability, relationships, self-esteem, etc.).

We can illustrate this with the case of a patient who showed good adjustment to her disease and did not feel hopeless about the future, but nevertheless had depressive symptoms that responded to behavioural interventions.

Betty was a 60-year-old retired office worker with stage 3 ovarian cancer. She underwent a successful course of treatment, but relapsed 3 years later. She made a good response to her second course of treatment, but was left with persistent tiredness, early morning wakening, and tearfulness. She made a slight improvement on antidepressant medication from her general practitioner, but was still significantly depressed when she was referred for psychiatric help.

As a consequence of her depressed mood, Betty's behavioural repertoire was greatly diminished. She was no longer doing many of the activities that she had previously enjoyed. This was exacerbated by the fact that she and her husband had moved into a bungalow just before the recurrence of her tumour. Much of the unpacking and decorating had consequently been left undone. Her negative automatic thoughts were self-critical: 'I shouldn't be like this, I ought to be able to get myself out of it' and 'I'm ashamed of myself for not doing these things about the house.'

She was resentful about moving home: 'Everything's gone wrong since I moved' and 'I wouldn't have got cancer again if I hadn't moved.'

She was trapping herself with her resentment, because it reduced her motivation to do anything in the new house. However, her inactivity led to further negative thoughts about her failure to act like her old self.

Betty was treated with CBT in combination with antidepressant medication. The homework assignment for the first week required her to monitor her activities and to start with some small activities (specifically in this case doing half an hour's knitting a day, and clearing three sections of the wardrobe) as a start to tidying her home. This produced an improvement in her mood in the course of a week. She recorded the amount of mastery she gained from each activity, and also graded each activity for pleasure. As is often the case, once she started to gain rewards from her behaviour, her motivation increased and she did more than she had set out to do (see Table 8.2).

Her mood continued to improve over the next few weeks, but her tiredness persisted, and she was admitted to hospital a few weeks later with abdominal pains. She was found to be suffering from acute myeloid leukaemia secondary to the treatment that she received for her ovarian cancer, and she died within a short time.

This case raises some interesting questions. First, was the patient's depression due to incipient leukaemia? Although this possibility cannot be excluded, her mood had been low for several weeks before the onset of any physical symptoms, and had perhaps been present as much as 3 months earlier, when she was still receiving treatment. Whatever the cause of her depression, it responded to psychological treatment within a short time period.

Secondly, was it appropriate to treat this patient with APT? If one had known that her lifespan was so short, the specific form of treatment that was used might not have been chosen. However, as is frequently the case, the physical condition of the patient changed during the course of therapy, and thus required new considerations and plans. The therapist needs to make judgements on the basis of the evidence available from the medical staff who are treating the patient. In CBT, problems are formulated as hypotheses. For example, the therapist will usually say 'Your tiredness and fatigue do not seem to be caused by any physical symptoms, but could well be a sign of depression. Perhaps we can work on your mood, and we'll see what happens to your tiredness.' This is in fact what happened. Betty's tiredness improved a little, but did not disappear completely.

Finally, this case example demonstrates the application of a graded task assignment approach. The tasks that were set were initially very simple and undemanding. As Betty's mood improved, the therapist helped her to choose more difficult and complex activities. Table 8.2 shows how she gradually increased the time she spent knitting from 35 minutes to 1 hour over the course of a week.

Summary

Behavioural interventions can provide a very effective means of challenging negative attitudes, providing a sense of personal control, and teaching

Table 8.2 Weekly activity schedule for a depressed patient with ovarian cancer, with activities graded for mastery (M) and pleasure (P)

Time	Monday	Tuesday	Wednesday	Thursday	Friday	Saturday	Sunday
9–10 a.m.							
10–11 a.m.							
11 a.m. – 12 noon		Discussed plans for new kitchen units (M10, P5)			Did knitting for 45 minutes (M10, P5)		
12–1 p.m.		Did knitting for 35 minutes (M10, P4)	Did ironing for 30 minutes		Did housework for 45 minutes (M10, P5)		
1–2 p.m.		Tidied section of wardrobe (M8, P3)				Shopping (M9, P5)	
2–3 p.m.							
3–4 p.m.			Visited friend (M10, P4)	Went shopping (M10, P4)			Friend's birthday (P6)
4–5 p.m.							
5–6 p.m.							
6–7 p.m.		Visited friend for a meal (M10, P6)				Prepared evening meal (M10, P5)	
7–8 p.m.				Did knitting for 35 minutes (M10, P5)			Did knitting for 1 hour (P6)
8–12 p.m.			Did knitting for 35 minutes (M10, P3)			Did knitting for 50 minutes (P6)	

self-help methods. They are usually the strategy of choice at the beginning of CBT. Behavioural experiments can be useful at any time during the course of therapy. When setting homework assignments, the following factors should be considered:

1. Tailor the assignment to the patient's needs. Wherever possible, set the task collaboratively and include the patient's partner.

2. Explain the rationale for each behavioural task, and obtain feedback on this.

3. Make homework tasks as specific and concrete as possible. Write them down for the patient to take away. Make clear predictions about what results are expected.

4. Make the task appropriate to the patient's level of education and their physical and psychological ability.

5. Try to create a 'no-lose' situation. Whenever possible, make sure that the patient will succeed at the task.

6. At the next session, ask for feedback on the effects of the task.

Chapter 9

Cognitive techniques I: Basic cognitive techniques

APT aims to give patients relief from emotional distress and to change maladaptive adjustment. Cognitive techniques constitute one of the most important sets of treatment strategies in therapy, and form a major component of the second phase of therapy. This chapter covers the following topics:

- the application of cognitive techniques, with special reference to the Dysfunctional Thought Record (DTR), which is the most commonly used format for identifying and challenging negative thoughts

- how to use the DTR to elicit, monitor, and evaluate thoughts and beliefs, and how to devise action plans

- five basic methods for evaluating thoughts and beliefs (reality testing, searching for alternatives, reattribution, decatastrophizing, and weighing up advantages and disadvantages)

- four further cognitive techniques (distraction, self-instructional training, cognitive rehearsal, and the use of imagery).

The application of cognitive techniques

Eliciting automatic thoughts and beliefs

The first step in any cognitive intervention is to identify the thoughts or beliefs that are relevant to the problem which is being presented. Once the problem that the patient wants to address in the session has been clarified, the therapist starts to explore the thoughts, feelings, behaviours, and physical sensations associated with it (see Figure 2.3 in Chapter 2). Understanding the way in which cognition shapes how we feel and what we do is central to the whole enterprise of therapy, and the process of helping the patient to see the link between thoughts, emotions, and behaviours is known as socialization into the model. At this stage it may be helpful to list the patient's experience of the problem under those four headings. Thus, for a patient who is worried about fatigue, the relevant features might be as follows:

Physical sensations	Thoughts	Feelings	Behaviours
Tiredness	'I can't do anything now'	Depressed	Withdraw, do less.
	'I'm useless'	Hopeless	

The cognitive model suggests that the way in which the person views their fatigue will have a significant impact on how they cope with it. The most reliable method of discovering the meaning of a symptom like this for the individual is through the thoughts that he or she reports about it. Reported thoughts (e.g. 'I hate myself') or images (e.g. 'I can see the cancer eating me up') are more valuable than the therapist's interpretations of what the patient might or ought to be feeling. In this context, a cognition is defined as 'a thought or a visual image that you may not be aware of unless you focus your attention on it.' The thoughts may therefore not be immediately apparent, but may need some practice before the person can identify what is upsetting them.

Beck et al (1979) recommend five steps that should be followed when teaching the patient to observe and record thoughts:

1. Define automatic thoughts.
2. Demonstrate the relationship between thoughts and feelings (or behaviour) using specific examples.
3. Demonstrate the presence of cognition from the patient's recent experience.
4. Assign homework for the patient to collect their thoughts.
5. Review the patient's thought records and provide concrete feedback.

There are several ways in which cognitions can be demonstrated to the patient.

1. The patient may be asked whether they had any thoughts about the therapy just before the session. For example, they may think 'This won't be of any use', 'I'm not mad – why are they sending me to a psychiatrist?', or 'I'm too far gone to be helped.'
2. The therapist can comment on any change in emotion during the session (e.g. the patient becoming tearful, appearing worried, etc.). These emotional changes often reveal 'hot cognitions' about the therapist or the therapy (e.g. 'I saw you look at your watch and I thought you weren't interested in what I was saying').

3. The patient is asked to remember the last time they experienced a strong emotion. A mental action replay of the situation, step by step, can reveal the thoughts or images that occurred at the time.

4. A recent experience can be re-created in the session through role play or imagery, and the patient can then be asked 'What's going through your mind right now?'

These techniques can be used in any session throughout therapy for eliciting thoughts about crucial events. When eliciting thoughts the therapist should try to establish the various meanings that the situation had for the individual. As many thoughts as possible should be identified, rather than stopping after the first one or two, because the first thoughts to be described may be fairly superficial. Asking yourself whether you would feel this upset if you thought this way can give a clue to whether the 'hot cognition' has been found. In addition to discussing thoughts in the session, the patient is encouraged to start monitoring their thoughts between sessions. When they have grasped the concept of automatic thoughts it is vital that they start to notice these thoughts in everyday life, and then find ways to evaluate them.

Monitoring automatic thoughts

Once the patient is familiar with the idea that thoughts are connected with emotional distress, the next step is to start recording these thoughts. The patient is given the automatic thought record (see Appendix 4) and asked to recall the negative thoughts that they had, together with the situation in which they occurred and the emotion that was felt. The instructions given will depend on the particular problems. For example, a patient who is depressed might be asked to write down their thoughts every time the depression gets worse. A woman who has an anxious preoccupation with cancer might be asked to recall the thoughts she has every time she starts to worry about a particular bodily symptom. Other patients can write down their thoughts on particular themes, such as hopelessness or unpredictability. Finally, if the problem is situational (e.g. hospital phobia or conditioned nausea), the patient can monitor the thoughts which occur in that particular situation. Specific guidance on what to record and when to do it will increase the likelihood that the homework assignment will be completed.

In our example of the patient who feels very tired, the homework could be to record those times when they feel tired (rating the symptom on a scale of 0–10), and then to record the thoughts and feelings that were experienced at the time.

People often need instruction and practice to record their automatic thoughts in the correct form. Some useful tips are listed below:

1. *Keep it brief*: 'I'm a failure' rather than 'I was walking home last night and he said something to me which made me feel terrible, and it was just like being told I had failed.'

2. *Distinguish clearly between situations, emotions, and thoughts*: The example in (1) above mixed them all up.

3. *Write statements rather than questions*: 'I can't think of anything I can do to help' rather than 'What am I going to do?'

4. *Write automatic thoughts separately*: Do not record them in a long diary in a stream-of-consciousness format.

5. *Make sure you really have got the automatic thought*. Many people write down reality-based statements such as 'We're in debt', but leave out the subsequent thoughts which are the ones that are really disturbing, such as 'I'm sure they're going to take us to court', 'I can't stand the shame', and 'I'm too ill to be able to cope.'

It is best if the patient records the thoughts at the time when they occurred, but this is not always possible. It may be necessary to set aside 15 minutes every night to write them down. When thought monitoring is being set as home-work, it should be reviewed at the beginning of each session.

At this stage the patient is not being asked to evaluate the thoughts. Just recording them is sometimes sufficient to reduce their frequency.

Evaluating automatic thoughts and beliefs

Once the concept of automatic thoughts has been grasped and the patient has successfully started to record them, the next step is to challenge them. Because people often describe a large number of thoughts, it is important to help them to find the best thought to challenge. One way of doing this is to take the thought which seems to explain most of the emotional response (i.e. the thought which is most upsetting), and to call this the 'hot thought' which the person needs to test. When the thoughts are identified and recorded they can initially be examined for cognitive distortions. Some examples are given below.

Automatic thought	*distortion*
'My husband doesn't make love to me any more.'	Arbitrary inference:
'I'm not attractive.'	
'No one can love me now I have cancer.'	Overgeneralization.

Finding the distortion can be the first step in demonstrating that the thought is unrealistic. Patients may find a handout that describes cognitive distortions helpful at this stage of therapy. One such handout for cancer patients is included in Appendix 2 of this book. The next step is to complete the alternative response column in the thought record. This is not an easy process, because it involves learning a new way of approaching thoughts and feelings. It is best to complete at least one thought record with the patient before they try to complete one as homework. Some methods of challenging negative thoughts will be described later. When thinking of alternative responses to thoughts in the thought record, the patient must make them personally meaningful. A common mistake is to use weak arguments, such as simply stating the opposite of the automatic thought. For instance, a woman with breast cancer might say 'No one can love me now' (automatic thought), to which 'People can love me' is the rational response. However, a more effective response might be 'I know my husband still finds me attractive because he tells me. I'm mixing up love and sexual attractiveness. My children love me, my husband loves me.' Table 9.1 shows how a thought record can be used to work with symptoms of fatigue, hopelessness, and depression.

Answers work best if they are specific and based on clearly described and testable occurrences. Table 9.2 summarizes the questions that patients can ask themselves when trying to evaluate negative thoughts.

Devising an action plan

Completion of a thought record will be more effective if the outcome is some definite action. If a convincing alternative to the thought is found, this can be used as a flashcard for dealing with the thought in the future. The patient can decide to rehearse how to interpret the situation differently when it next occurs. A behavioural task often suggests itself from the exercise. In Table 9.1 the fatigued patient came up with two ways of dealing with feeling low because he could not play with his 3-year-old granddaughter. First, he could think of less physical activities they could do together, and secondly he could wait until one of the days when he felt less tired and invite her round then. Challenging the negative thoughts allows you to be more constructive in your problem solving. In many cases a plan of action becomes obvious from the results of the thought record. If the patient is still unsure whether the negative thought is accurate or not, a behavioural experiment (see Chapter 8) can be arranged to test it. In Table 9.1 the patient decided to try making the bed regularly as an experiment to test whether his tiredness was entirely physical, or whether it was perhaps a symptom of his depression.

Table 9.1 Thought record of a patient with fatigue, hopelessness, and depression

Situation	Fatigue (rate on a scale of 0–10)	Emotions (rate on a scale of 0–10)	Automatic thoughts	Alternative response	Action Plan
My granddaughter came and I felt too tired to play with her	8	Depressed Hopeless 10	I can't do anything now. I'm useless	I'm having a difficult time today. I'm more breathless than usual, but I can still play some less tiring games with her. Nobody else thinks I'm useless. I can still enjoy being with her even if we don't play hard	Plan games I can play in future that aren't too physical. Invite them round on days when I'm feeling less tired.
Trying to make the bed	6	Depressed 5	I'll never manage this. I'm useless. What's the point?	I did it yesterday, even though I felt very tired. I know that some of this tiredness is psychological, not physical. If I have a go. I'll feel better for at least trying	Don't give up immediately because I feel tired. Try it and see if I can do it.

Basic methods for evaluating thoughts and beliefs

The process of monitoring and testing automatic thoughts is basic to cognitive therapy. The techniques that the patient uses to challenge these thoughts are part of the problem-solving procedure demonstrated in the session. Once the problem has been defined, the associated negative emotions are acknowledged and the patient is encouraged to express them openly (see Chapter 7). Then the negative automatic thoughts are elicited and one or more of the cognitive interventions described below is employed to deal with the problem. This is frequently done with the help of a thought record, but on other occasions it may be done through more informal discussion.

Table 9.2 Questions that patients can ask themselves when evaluating negative automatic thoughts

1. What are my reasons for believing that this is true?
What are my reasons for *not* believing that this is true?
2. Are there other ways of looking at this?
Is there an alternative explanation?
What would I say to a friend if they were in this situation?
3. If it is true, is it really as bad as I fear?
What is the *worst* that could happen?
What is the *best* that could happen?
What is *most likely* to happen?
How can I cope with it?
4. What are the advantages of thinking in this way?
What are the disadvantages?

The techniques described here cover five of the commonest methods for testing thoughts and beliefs. These are:

1. reality testing
2. searching for alternatives
3. reattribution
4. decatastrophizing
5. weighing advantages and disadvantages.

The distinctions between these different techniques are useful for learning cognitive strategies, but they should not be regarded as hard-and-fast categories. As novice therapists become more experienced, they will find themselves using several different techniques within a short space of time in order to achieve cognitive change. All therapists develop their own individual techniques, which are not necessarily covered here.

Reality testing

Reality testing simply means testing the validity of a thought or belief. The patient is asked to look for the evidence that supports or does not support the belief.

Reality testing is one of the core cognitive procedures. The goal is to distinguish realistic sadness from depression, and to distinguish realistic fear from irrational anxiety. Cancer causes tremendous suffering in its own right, but we may increase this suffering when we buy into extreme or unhelpful thinking. Fear of recurrence is a good example of this. Everyone with cancer has to live with the constant possibility that the disease will return. For some individuals the likelihood of recurrence is relatively low, yet they find it difficult not to ruminate about it. Examining the evidence allows the patient to form an accurate opinion of how realistic the fears really are. In patients with early-stage disease and a good prognosis, reality testing helps to promote a realistically optimistic view of the prognosis. Feelings of guilt, self-blame, worthlessness, and isolation are also often the result of distorted thinking:

'I will never get a job now that I've had cancer.'
'I'm going to die alone'
'There's nothing I can do about it.'

Skilful questioning draws out the fallacies in the patient's beliefs. When looking for evidence, the therapist can draw on a variety of sources, including the following:

1. the patient's past experience
2. the patient's knowledge and observation of other people's behaviour and experience
3. reference to reputable sources of information (e.g. books, professionals, etc.)
4. reference to the patient's own standards
5. the rules of everyday logic.

Example 1

Let us consider the example of a woman who has recently had a colostomy and is afraid to attend social gatherings.

Step 1
Elicit automatic thoughts:

'I can't take the chance – I might smell.'
'I won't go – I'm so embarrassed.'
'They'd never want to see me again – I'd be so ashamed'.

Step 2
Identify the 'hot thought' that causes most distress:

'I can't take the chance – I might smell.'

Step 3
Look for the evidence for and against this belief.

1. *Using past experience*

   Has the patient attended any social events since the operation? Did anything happen to suggest that people noticed anything?

   If the response is yes, then on what did the patient base her judgement that someone noticed the smell? (This challenges distortion of arbitrary inferences.)

   Are there any alternative explanations for her interpretation that people noticed the smell? (This challenges the arbitrary inference.)

   How many people did she talk to who did not notice the smell, as opposed to those who did? (This challenges selective abstraction.)

2. *Using knowledge of other people*

   Has she asked people close to her whether there is a smell? From her knowledge of them, are they likely to be lying if they say no?

   From her knowledge of people, are they really likely to ostracize her if she does smell?

3. *Using information source*

   Could she find out from a stoma nurse whether this is a problem that she is likely to encounter?

4. *Using the patient's own standards*

   If she was in a similar situation, would she reject someone because they had a post-operative problem?

5. *Using logic*

   If she bases her assumptions on the fact that she can smell herself, how likely is it that other people can smell her?

These are all approaches that can be used to test this patient's assumption that there will be dire consequences if she attends a social event. After working on this with her, the therapist could set up a homework assignment where the patient tested the belief by going into a social situation to find out whether people do in fact notice anything. If the belief did prove to be true, the therapist could help the patient to use problem solving to find strategies for reducing the smell (e.g. consulting the stoma nurse for advice).

Example 2

This is an excerpt from a therapy session with a 43-year-old woman with breast cancer. On the Hospital Anxiety and Depression Scale (HADS) (Zigmond and Snaith, 1983) she had a score of 19 for anxiety and 2 for depression. On the Mental Adjustment to Cancer Scale (MACS) (Watson et al, 1988) she had a score of 34 (out of a possible maximum of 36) on the anxious preoccupation scale. This picture of predominant anxiety was supported by the patient's clinical state. Cancer represented a considerable threat to her personal domain. She had a strong belief that she could only be happy if she was sexually attractive, and she saw cancer as a threat to her attractiveness. Her doctors suggested that she should be treated with anti-oestrogen therapy. This suggestion 'terrorized' her with the thought of having an artificial menopause and ceasing to be desirable. The therapist used questioning to test the validity of her fear.

Patient: When I think of the menopause. I think what unknown terrors are there ahead?

It's unknown territory.

Therapist: Do you know any people who have been through the menopause and are still attractive?

Patient: Yes, I have one very good friend … but hers was an artificial menopause … she's 55.

Therapist: So that would be a menopause similar to the sort you might go through?

Patient: Yes.

Therapist: So you have evidence that it is possible for people to go through the menopause and to come out of it still attractive. Is she someone who still has an active sex life?

Patient: Oh yes, very much so.

Therapist: And does she say that she's been adversely affected by the menopause?

Patient: No – I mean, I haven't asked her in so many words, but I'm sure not, no.

Therapist: That's interesting, because what you're saying is that the menopause conjures up this feeling of terror of the unknown, but your friend's experience is that it was fairly benign.

Patient: Yes.

This intervention had the specific effect of challenging the patient's belief that there would be no sex life after the menopause. It also had the more general effect of introducing her to the idea that strongly held beliefs based purely on emotion might be fallacious. Thus the groundwork was laid for her to base her beliefs on evidence rather than on emotional reasoning.

Searching for alternatives

This technique involves exploring alternative ways of viewing the situation. As such it can be used as part of reality testing, but can also be used when the thoughts are likely to be realistic. If the person's negative thoughts are accurate, they may still be unhelpful, and there may be other ways of looking at the situation. People with negative styles of adjusting to cancer are locked into a mental set that limits their ability to see beyond a narrow range of options. The hopeless patient selectively focuses on the negative aspects of the future. By asking them to list alternative outcomes that might be possible, the therapist begins to overcome the pervasive negative thinking. At first the patient will only be able to think of negative options, but as the therapist presses them for more alternatives, the patient will find that the options become increasingly positive.

The effectiveness of this method can be increased if the patient writes down the ideas in a list. Putting one's thoughts on paper allows some distancing, and many people find that their negative thoughts look quite unrealistic when they are written down. This does not have to be limited to prediction of the future. A useful technique is to ask the patient and their partner to make a list of alternative ways of viewing themselves. A demoralized patient will initially come up with a list of weaknesses. The therapist can then say 'Now let's put down what you see as your strengths, next to your weaknesses.' This information can then become part of the treatment plan, which should include ways of building on the strengths of the patient and their partner.

Weaknesses

1. I worry too much.
2. I often feel unable to cope.
3. I rely too much on other people.

Strengths

1. I care about other people.
2. Once I make up my mind I stick to it.
3. I'm conscientious.
4. I'm reliable.

The weaknesses can also be the focus of attention, first to see whether the patient is distorting the facts or underselling him- or herself, and secondly, if the weaknesses that are listed appear to be accurate, they can be added to the agenda as problems to be solved.

The technique can also be applied to finding new ways of viewing cancer. The couple can brainstorm ways in which their lives might be changed for the better as a result of cancer (e.g. spending more time together, learning to take things easy, planning things they had always wanted to do, taking more care of their health). If they cannot think of anything, the exercise can be used as an opportunity to encourage them to plan ways of improving their lives. There is some evidence that patients who can see positive changes in their lives as a result of cancer show better psychological adjustment (Taylor et al, 1984; Tennen and Affleck, 1999), and that cognitive behavioural techniques can increase 'benefit finding' by cancer patients (Antoni et al, 2001).

Some changes for the better which patients have reported include the following:

1. 'We are closer together as a family.'
2. 'We value the time we have to get there.'
3. 'I find simple things more enjoyable.'
4. 'We don't argue about trivia.'
5. 'Life has more meaning now.'

Another way of looking for alternatives is to ask what you might say to a friend in a similar situation. People who are very hard on themselves about their appearance or functioning are usually much less critical when they look at others. Identifying this double standard can create some leverage in helping the patient to view him- or herself more compassionately. If necessary the therapist can role play an interaction with a friend to reinforce this alternative perspective.

Reattribution

Reattribution is a specific example of the alternatives method. We all try to find causal explanations for the things that happen to us. It is common for people with cancer to try to find someone to blame for their illness – either themselves or another person. A *responsibility pie chart* can be used to challenge unreasonable blame. For instance, a woman who blames herself for her teenage son's bad behaviour might be helped to identify various people and situations that might have some involvement in causing and solving the problem, including the following:

1. me
2. my son himself
3. his father
4. the teachers at school
5. the other children at school
6. the effect of the stress of cancer on the family.

Figure 9.1 shows how the initial response, which consisted of blaming herself 100% was tempered by placing other factors in the responsibility pie.

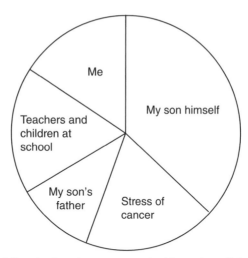

Fig. 9.1 Responsibility pie chart for a woman who blames herself for her son's bad behaviour.

Inevitably the person has to accept that they cannot be completely responsible for anyone else's behaviour.

Bodily symptoms can be another focus of misattributions. Patients with panic attacks tend to focus on the physical symptoms of anxiety, such as palpitations, and interpret them as a heart attack. Reattribution training involves getting them to look at other possible explanations for their experiences. Cancer patients with the anxious preoccupation style of adjustment also focus on minor physical symptoms as signs of a return of the disease. Changing the interpretation of the aches and pains is an important part of helping their anxiety.

Decatastrophizing

The anxious patient will predict the most threatening outcome of any situation, and will have vivid images of their prediction. They rarely go beyond this to think in more detail about the real consequences. However, by continually pursuing the patient with the question 'And what would happen next?', the therapist can arrive at the most feared consequence. Sometimes the person is able to see that what they fear is not really so bad after all. This process can be repeated using imagery, and often the images become progressively more realistic and less frightening.

The same procedure can be used for the more reality-based fears of people with cancer. If the anxious patient fears a recurrence, the most frightening type of recurrence can be rehearsed using imagery. Sometimes the patient can use the relaxation method while doing this. This does not attempt to make it a pleasant experience, but can help to show the person that it is an experience with which they might be able to cope.

A woman who had undergone a mastectomy for breast cancer was told by her doctor that the mammogram which was performed at a check-up showed some suspicious signs in the other breast, and he needed to repeat the test in 3 months' time. Although the patient put on a brave face, she was obviously very concerned. Exploring her fears allowed her to express her feelings of anger and despair openly. As she cried she was able to identify the thoughts that underlay her fears. These were not directly connected with death, but with the implications of treatment. She thought 'I won't be able to cope', 'I won't be able to stand it', and 'My boyfriend won't want me if I have to have another mastectomy.'

Once she had described her thoughts she was able to challenge them very quickly. She remembered that she had coped well before, and felt that she would find it easier now that she knew what was involved. She was also able to see that if this was indeed a recurrence, it had been found at an early stage and might not require a mastectomy. Her boyfriend had been very understanding in the past, and there was no problem with their sexual relationship, so it did not seem likely that he would suddenly reject her now.

Decatastrophizing did not falsely convince her that there was nothing to worry about. The thought of cancer recurring was frightening and undesirable, but it was a stress that she and her partner could cope with together. Fortunately, her next appointment did not confirm the suspicions, and she was given a clean bill of health.

Weighing advantages and disadvantages

A patient was determined that if she had to have chemotherapy she would not go to work and would stay at home all day. The therapist used questioning to establish what the advantages and disadvantages of this course of action would be:

Advantages	Disadvantages
I would have time to prepare the Bristol diet (but I had 3 weeks off recently and I didn't do it then)	I'd miss out on a lot of things
	I don't like being alone
	I would not be getting on with daily life

The benefits and costs of a course of action can be written down and the patient then asked to decide whether one outweighs the other. As a further step, the patient can rate each item for importance. This will give a rough estimate of the extent to which one option outweighs the other. This technique can prove useful when dealing with thoughts about whether to go through with a course of treatment.

Other cognitive techniques

Distraction

Patients who are coping often selectively attend to aspects of their world that they can still control, rather than dwelling on the areas where they can no longer exert any influence. Patients with negative adjustment are plagued by automatic thoughts and selectively attend to negative aspects of the environment, so anything that changes the focus of their attention may be of use as an initial coping strategy. However, there is always a danger that these methods can become safety-seeking behaviours that give false reassurance and even prevent the patient from testing their negative thoughts. A person with an anxious preoccupation may be continually monitoring their bodily symptoms (e.g. a lumpectomy patient may be examining her breasts daily). A vicious circle is set up when non-pathological physical sensations are misinterpreted, causing further anxiety and further compulsive self-examination. This is similar to the selective attention to bodily sensations that is observed in health anxiety (Salkovskis and Warwick, 1986). In these cases distraction may be able to break into the spiral of increasing anxiety by interrupting the excessive focus on somatic sensations.

Distracting procedures include the following:

1. focusing on the immediate surroundings and describing them in detail, aloud if possible

2. engaging someone in conversation, which may help to relieve the panicky feelings associated with treatment procedures

3. performing a mental exercise (e.g. mental arithmetic, reciting a poem).

It is our experience that these techniques are most effective if, rather than being used to avoid a negative experience, they are conceptualized as steps towards a valued goal. One patient who faced several courses of intravenous chemotherapy was keen to continue to learn Portuguese, so she decided that she would bring her MP3 player with her and listen to Portuguese language tapes during the treatment. In this way she not only took her mind off the distressing experience, but also engaged in a pleasurable and constructive activity towards a goal that was important to her.

Many of the behavioural techniques can therefore be used to help patients to distract themselves from negative automatic thoughts. Because of the risk that distraction may become avoidance, the therapist should use this method with caution, and will usually want to help the patient to address their fears directly, to prove that they are not as catastrophic as he or she believes.

Self-instructions

Meichenbaum (1977, 1985) developed the use of self-instructions to facilitate task performance and to provide a means of coping with stress. Patients can be taught to prepare things that they can say to themselves in times of stress. These should be developed by the patient him- or herself, and not imposed by the therapist. For instance, a woman with a lung secondary that causes occasional dyspnoea may initially monitor her negative thoughts as follows:

Feeling breathless: 'I'll never get better.'

The patient and the therapist then collaborate to find self-statements that promote a constructive coping style. Whenever the patient feels breathless she can use this as a cue for more helpful self-talk, as shown below.

Coping self-statements

'I know the chemotherapy is shrinking my lump.'
　'This isn't going to ruin my life.'
　This form of coping strategy can be expanded to include a whole plan for coping. One patient who was continually troubled by fears of the disease returning developed a four-step plan of action:

1. Take a deep breath.
2. Look again (i.e. confront the pain, skin blemish, etc.).
3. Should I be worrying?
4. Reward myself for coping.

She wrote these instructions down on a small card and kept it in her purse so that she could review them whenever she felt under stress. These coping self-statements can be helpful when it is not possible or desirable to complete a full thought record. If the patient has completed several thought records and the same thoughts keep recurring, they can simply write down the alternative, more balanced thoughts on a flashcard for easy reference. Not everyone is able to use thought records, in which case it is perfectly acceptable for the therapist and the patient to test thoughts together during the session, and to collaborate on the construction of a set of answers to the negative thoughts, which the patient can then use outside the session.

Cognitive rehearsal

Problem solving is an important part of therapy, and once a solution to a problem has been found, it may be worth rehearsing the new coping strategies during the session. Sometimes this may involve role play, whereas at other times a purely cognitive rehearsal may be appropriate. The patient can rehearse using imagery of the problem and the proposed coping strategy. This technique often produces further automatic thoughts about how the strategy might not work, which can then be addressed. Applications include getting ready for a medical appointment, coping with treatment, etc. The case example described in the section on cognitive interventions for patients with anxious preoccupation (see p. 145) demonstrates the use of this method to prepare parents to tell their daughter about her mother's diagnosis of cancer.

Imagery techniques

Cognitive rehearsal is only one of the many uses of imagery in cognitive therapy. Three possible applications for people with cancer are exposure in imagination, imagery modification, and visualization.

Exposure in imagination

Patients who are phobic or who have conditioned anticipatory nausea can imagine the aversive stimulus while they are relaxed. Although this method is less effective than exposure *in vivo*, it may be necessary when real-life exposure is not possible. In the classical systematic desensitization procedure, the patient relaxes and imagines increasingly frightening scenes (a hierarchy of frightening situations is constructed beforehand). Each time the patient becomes anxious they go back to relaxation until the anxiety is under control.

Image modification

Many images can be identified in people under stress. Depressed cancer patients are more likely to experience intrusive images of past events (often memories of illness, injury, or death) (Brewin et al, 1998). These images are cognitions, and as such can be dealt with using the same cognitive techniques that we have described for automatic thoughts. Identifying the distortion in the image can help to generate ideas about how the image can be changed. Once the distortion has been found, the patient needs to think about how to modify the image to demonstrate that the meaning behind it is untrue. For instance, a woman with a successfully treated sarcoma reported anxiety associated with images of herself as a child. She had been seriously ill when she was 11 years old, and the cancer reactivated memories of herself as a helpless, dependent invalid. In order to remind herself that these were images from the past, not facts about the present or the future, she altered the picture of herself alone in hospital by imagining putting on her clothes and leaving. Images that seem vivid and real can be modified by putting them on a mental television screen and visualizing oneself watching them with a friend or family member. This helps to create distance, puts them in perspective, and reinforces the idea that they are mental constructs, not perceptions. Unpleasant images can be changed a little at a time until the whole scene is transformed. People differ greatly in the extent to which they can use these procedures, but if images form a significant part of their cognitive content it is worth experimenting with some of these techniques.

Visualization

Some patients wish to find ways in which they can fight cancer themselves, and may ask about the methods that are sometimes referred to as visualization. This can be used as part of APT if it seems appropriate for the individual. More detailed descriptions of this method have been provided by Simonton et al (1978) and Borysenko et al (1986).

The patient goes into a relaxed state and then conjures up an image of the cancer being destroyed by the treatment and the body's defences. In the image the cancer is composed of weak and ineffectual cells that are destroyed and cleared by the body's white blood cells. The treatment is visualized as a friendly, helpful process that kills the cancer cells. The images can be whatever the patient chooses (e.g. the white cells can be visualized as fish eating the cancer, or knights on white horses). At the end of the session the patient gives him- or herself a mental pat on the back for participating in his or her own recovery. This exercise should be practised for 10 to 15 minutes a day. Simonton et al (1978) recommend that is should be practiced three times a day, but this may not be practicable for most people.

The significant points about imagery can be summarized as follows:

1. The cancer cells are weak and confused.
2. The treatment is strong and powerful.
3. The healthy cells have no difficulty in repairing any slight damage that the treatment might cause.
4. The army of white blood cells is vast, and overwhelms the cancer cells.
5. The white blood cells are aggressive, eager for battle, and quick to seek out the cancer cells and destroy them.
6. The dead cancer cells are flushed from the body normally and naturally.

7. By the end of the imagery, the patient imagines him- or herself healthy and free of cancer.

8. The patient sees him- or herself reaching his or her goals in life.

(adapted from Simonton et al, 1978).

Not all patients take to this method. Many find it frustrating trying to imagine the tumour shrinking when they know that in fact it is not changing in size. However, for some individuals this approach can be very effective in instilling a sense of control. Visual images of the cancer and its treatment can often be used in other ways, without necessarily incorporating the whole Simonton method. Valuable information is obtained by asking for imagery. For example, one patient who dreaded chemotherapy reported seeing a large neon sign that said *POISON*. Using the visualization method allowed her to view the treatment completely differently – as a strong helper – to the extent that she wished to continue chemotherapy even when the medical staff felt it was no longer proving effective. Another patient described an image of chemotherapy as a monster. This vivid metaphor could be used in therapy, and a number of cognitive techniques were needed to challenge her fears. These approaches must only be used with patients who basically wish to have drug treatment but are fearful of it. Trying to convince patients to have chemotherapy against their will is not a function of APT.

Table 9.3 Cognitive and behavioural techniques

Technique	Implementation
Behavioural techniques	Relaxation
	Graded task assignment
	Planning for the future
	Behavioural experiments
Cognitive coping strategies	Self-instructions
	Distraction
	Cognitive rehearsal
Cognitive restructuring *Surface*	Thought monitoring
	Identifying cognitive distortions
	Reality testing
	Searching for alternatives
	Decatastrophizing
	Weighing advantages and disadvantages
Deep	Making explicit underlying fears, assumptions, rules, and core beliefs

Summary

The cognitive rationale is explained during the first session, and cognitive techniques are introduced in the second or third session. Simple cognitive techniques can be used as coping strategies, but it is usually necessary to restructure thoughts. Monitoring and challenging negative automatic thoughts is the key procedure, and the patient is encouraged to undertake this as homework. Table 9.3 lists some of the common behavioural and cognitive techniques that are used in therapy.

Chapter 10

Cognitive techniques II: Working with anxiety and depression

In the previous chapter we introduced the basic cognitive techniques and illustrated their use. In this chapter we shall consider the application of these techniques to anxiety and depression.

We shall describe the following:

- ◆ cognitive interventions for patients with anxious preoccupation
- ◆ how to deal with fear of recurrence
- ◆ cognitive interventions for helpless/hopeless patients
- ◆ a case example of CBT in action.

Cognitive interventions for patients with anxious preoccupation

Fear of recurrence is common following the diagnosis and treatment of cancer. For instance, more than 50% of women who have undergone curative treatment for breast cancer have moderate to high levels of fear of recurrence (van den Beuken-van Everdingen et al, 2008), while one-third of head and neck cancer patients have high levels of fear of recurrence (Llewellyn et al, 2008). In anxious preoccupation the focus is on the danger posed by the risk of recurrence or disease progression. The person becomes hypervigilant with regard to any potential threat from the disease, to the extent that normal physical symptoms may be misinterpreted as signs of cancer. The patient feels unable to control the situation, and underestimates the coping strategies and rescue factors that are available. Finally, the objective prognosis is uncertain. The preoccupied patient frantically looks around for ways to control the disease and make the future more predictable (e.g. by seeking reassurance, obtaining more information, removing all causes of stress, or trying alternative treatments). The following case example shows how cognitive techniques were used with an anxious patient. The reader can assess how the cognitive components of the survival schema were addressed during therapy. As an exercise, the reader might also note down which cognitive techniques were used.

Mrs W, aged 39 years, was referred by her medical oncologist who wrote:

> Her main problem is that she is finding it extremely difficult to come to terms with the fact that she has cancer and may die from it. At present she finds she cannot reconcile herself to either of these positions, and although I have stressed that we are not in a situation yet where all treatment has failed, it is naturally a realistic fear, and I have not tried to hide this fact from her. She herself has requested formal psychological assessment and counselling.

Mrs W noticed a swelling on her neck which was found to be due to a secondary anaplastic carcinoma, probably arising from the lung. She and her husband were fully and sensitively informed of the diagnosis by her oncologist. Treatment with adriamycin, cyclophosphamide and etoposide produced tumour regression but was accompanied by unpleasant side-effects, namely fatigue, nausea, vomiting, and alopecia. The patient was referred for psychiatric consultation after she had completed chemotherapy. Her general practitioner had prescribed triazolam for her anxiety, without noticeable effect. Mrs W was the only child of middle-aged parents. She described her childhood as happy. There was no family history or previous personal history of psychiatric illness, but she had always been a rather anxious person with some perfectionist tendencies. She had never had any serious physical illness. She had done reasonably well at school and became a medical laboratory technician, working for 10 years in one hospital. She left her job to get married at the age of 26 years. Her husband was a stockbroker, and they had one daughter, aged 12 years, who had become 'rebellious and difficult' since her mother's illness. The marriage was described by both partners as 'close and happy.' They had many friends, and until Mrs W's illness they had led an active social life. For the last three years she had worked for a charity.

At interview, the patient was found to be moderately depressed and severely anxious. There was no diurnal variation in her mood, nor was there any evidence of suicidal ideas. She complained that all of her usual activities and interests had become overshadowed by constant fear of dying and uncertainty about the future. She felt that she had no control over her life and that she was unable to plan ahead. Her husband confirmed her story, adding that she frequently examined her body for signs of cancer and continually asked for reassurance. She was well motivated for psychological therapy, and her husband agreed to participate.

The patient and her husband were seen together for two sessions, followed by three sessions with the patient alone. The principal problems identified were as follows:

1. pervasive anxiety
2. lack of control over the patient's life, and inability to plan ahead

3. preoccupation with recurrence of cancer and dying

4. difficulty in dealing with her rebellious daughter.

It was decided to begin with relaxation training in an attempt to reduce the patient's anxiety. This proved unsuccessful. However, Mrs W rapidly learned how to identify and challenge negative automatic thoughts. As she began to challenge her negative thoughts with alternative responses, her husband observed that she was becoming less anxious. The therapist suggested that her anxiety was related to her negative automatic thoughts, and that it could therefore be brought under control by the patient herself. When Mrs W found that she could indeed reduce her anxiety by challenging her negative thoughts, she also began to feel more in control, which in turn further reduced her anxiety. She was then encouraged to plan daily activities that could give her pleasure and a sense of mastery. She began by inviting a friend round for coffee, resuming work and (more difficult) attempting to stop triazolam (see Table 10.1).

During the second session, the issue of her daughter's rebellious behaviour was discussed with Mrs W and her husband. It transpired that the daughter's change in behaviour coincided with the commencement of chemotherapy. The parents had not informed their daughter of the diagnosis, in order to 'protect' her.

Table 10.1 Record of Mrs W's automatic thoughts

Situation	Emotion	Automatic thoughts	Alternative response
Tidying up	Anxious (50%)	I've been having my period for 2 weeks. What if I have cancer of the ovary? (50%)	It's probably the therapy. Body scans didn't reveal a problem with the ovaries (100%)
Sitting on the sofa – shoulder is hurting	Anxious (60%)	My shoulder is hurting – the tumour hasn't gone (60%)	The tumour has not disappeared completely – *yet*. The pain is much less and I have not taken any painkillers for 2 days (100%)
My daughter woke up with a backache	Fear (100%)	What if she has a brain tumour? (70%)	It is most likely she has some kind of virus, or that it's psychosomatic (90%)
In bed, trying to relax	Very sad and anxious (70%)	I only believe I will go into remission because I can't face the alternative (my death) (60%)	I have every reason to be optimistic because: I feel better the tumour is responding to treatment. I am *beginning* to accept my mortality

The therapist asked the parents to consider the possibility that their daughter's difficult behaviour was a reaction to being kept in the dark about her mother's illness. The advantages and disadvantages of telling their daughter the correct diagnosis were examined. Eventually, Mrs W and her husband decided to tell their daughter the truth. In the remainder of the session they rehearsed with the therapist precisely what they would say to their daughter. This course of action had the desired effect. Their daughter took the news calmly at first, then became angry because they had lied to her and made her feel excluded, and finally her acting-out behaviour ceased as she became more affectionate towards her mother.

During the remaining three sessions, Mrs W consolidated the gains that she had made. She and her daughter became much closer, and her self-esteem increased as she found that her daughter needed her. She returned part-time to her previous charity work, and began to see friends again. Her anxious preoccupation with cancer receded. The fear of dying remained, but this could now be discussed openly and realistically. The patient faced the prospect that her lifespan was likely to be considerably reduced. The last negative automatic thoughts (see Table 10.1) showed that she was beginning to accept her mortality. Based on the premise that her life would be shortened and that it was therefore vital to make the most of that life, Mrs W and the therapist drew up plans to make Mrs W's remaining life as rewarding and pleasurable as possible.

At the end of therapy, Mrs W was no longer anxious, she felt in control again, and her relationship with her daughter had improved greatly. At a 4-month follow-up it emerged that Mrs W had undergone a course of radiotherapy, and her cancer was now in a state of remission. Psychologically, she maintained the gains that she had made (see Table 10.2).

The cognitive techniques described in this example included the following:

1. *monitoring and challenging automatic thoughts*
2. *reality testing* (realistic versus unrealistic fears about the future)
3. *searching for alternatives (reattribution)* in the patient's thought diary
4. *weighing advantages and disadvantages* with regard to telling the patient's daughter about the cancer
5. *cognitive rehearsal* of how the couple would tell their daughter about the cancer.

The behavioural techniques that were used included the following:

1. relaxation
2. activity scheduling
3. planning for the future.

Table 10.2 Case report: Mrs W

Assessment measures	Before APT	After APT	4-month follow-up
Mental Adjustment to Cancer Scale (MACS)	40	51	50
Fighting spirit	14	7	8
Hopelessness	31	17	18
Anxious preoccupation	18	19	20
Fatalism			
Hospital Anxiety and Depression Scale (HADS)	11	6	6
Depression	17	8	9
Anxiety			

In anxious preoccupation, the patient's sensitivity to the possibility of recurrence often leads to heightened awareness of bodily sensations, repetitive scanning of the sensations, and misattribution of these to cancer.

The attribution 'It must be in my bones' causes more anxiety and tension. The patient now focuses all of their attention on the physical symptoms, magnifying their sensations and thus producing further anxiety (see Figure 10.1). Anxious patients frequently use safety-seeking behaviours (Salkovskis, 1991). These are attempts to escape or mitigate the consequence of their fears, which may give relief in the short term, but which in the longer term are often maladaptive. Figure 10.1 shows how selective attention leads to the safety behaviour of checking for signs of recurrence. The more the patient checks for these

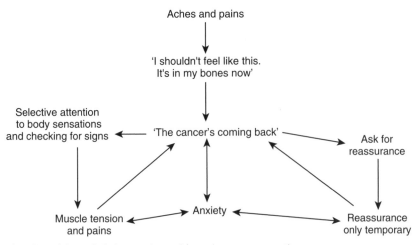

Fig. 10.1 Vicious circle in a patient with anxious preoccupation.

signs, the more she reminds herself of her fears. In addition, the physical act of checking (e.g. by palpating the armpit for signs of lymph nodes) in itself causes discomfort and pain, and this further increases anxiety. Another common safety behaviour is reassurance seeking. When she obtains reassurance from her partner or the doctor the patient temporarily feels better, but then doubts set in and the need for reassurance returns. It is best to help the patient to come to their own understanding of how these behaviours contribute to the maintenance of anxiety, so the therapist uses guided discovery and Socratic questioning to demonstrate the effects of the vicious circle. This is particularly important for people who are facing adversity, as the cognitive model can appear overly rational if it is simply imposed on the patient through psychoeducation (Moorey, 2011). Once the patient can see that her thoughts and behaviours may be contributing to her anxiety, the next step is to set up behavioural experiments to test the safety behaviours. The patient could decide to spend two days attending more closely to the symptoms and checking for them, followed by two days without checking, and then decide which method produced less distress and physical symptoms. Similarly, an experiment can be devised in which the patient spends some time asking her partner for reassurance, followed by some time resisting this urge and evaluating the effect. It may be important in these circumstances to ensure that the partner does not give in to the often insistent and persuasive attempts of an anxious patient to get him to reassure her that everything is all right. An excellent resource on the use of behavioural experiments is the *Oxford Guide to Behavioural Experiments in Cognitive Therapy* (Bennett-Levy et al, 2004).

Cognitive techniques can also be helpful in relation to the patient's fear of being unable to control the situation. The therapist can help the patient to look for evidence of how they have been in control of other areas of their life. Here again the focus shifts from cancer to life. The partner can be brought in to remind the patient of their strengths. Similar techniques can be employed for dealing with uncertainty and the fear of recurrence.

Reality testing

How likely is recurrence?
Is the time spent worrying proportional to the risk of the recurrence?

Alternatives

Are there any alternative outcomes?
Why not assume the best prognosis possible with your type of illness?

Decatastrophizing

What's the worst that could happen?

Since fear of recurrence is such a common problem among patients with cancer, some kind of scheme for approaching it can help the therapist. We have found the following broad plan useful when dealing with patients who have difficulty coping with uncertainty about their prognosis.

General strategy for dealing with fear of recurrence

1. Use the best prognosis available from the patient's doctor.
2. Modify the approach according to the prognosis:

    (a) *No sign of active disease*:

    If the patient is considered to be disease-free, encourage a search for alternative statements to 'I've got cancer' (e.g. 'I had cancer, but all the evidence suggests that it has gone').

    (b) *Active disease*:

    If treatment might bring about a remission, help the patient to focus on and work towards this. If success is unlikely, use cognitive, behavioural, and acceptance strategies (see below and Chapter 14).

Worry

Worry is a very understandable reaction to having cancer and is to some degree normal, especially during times of uncertainty (e.g. when waiting for the results of tests, or when the date of a check-up is approaching). However, for a significant number of patients it can become a major problem. Research on worry in the setting of generalized anxiety disorder has proliferated in the last decade, and a number of features of worry have become clearer (Dugas and Robichaud, 2007). Worry is often perceived as having both positive and negative qualities (Wells, 2000). People can have positive beliefs about worry. These may be concerned with the need to be prepared:

> 'If I don't prepare myself I won't be able to cope.'
> 'I must think of every possibility.'
> 'I have to try everything I can think of to get better.'

Alternatively, they may be associated with a superstitious fear that being positive may be tempting fate:

> 'If I don't worry the cancer might come back.'
> 'I daren't think of a good outcome because I'll be devastated if I get bad news.'

However, people can also have negative beliefs about the effect that worry has on their lives:

'The worry may bring my cancer on again.'
'The stress of worry will make me more ill.'
'Worry is uncontrollable.'
'I'll go mad with worry.'

Beliefs about the usefulness of worry as a problem-solving tool are associated with the perpetuation of worry cycles. In effective problem solving the person identifies a problem, explores solutions, chooses one, and then tries it out before evaluating it. However, when we worry we get into cognitive loops. For instance, we may be facing the possibility that a test result will show disease spread. We may look at different treatment options available to us but know that until we get the news and discuss these options with our doctor we cannot come to any definite conclusion. At this point we might feel very uncomfortable with not knowing what the best course of treatment would be, so we might think through all the options again, seeking more information, checking what our partner thinks, and trying to imagine all of the different permutations. Once we are in the worry cycle it becomes difficult to escape the loop. With every possible solution another 'What if?' question arises and we start the whole process again.

Further factors that maintain worry are no longer feeling in control, and feeling unable to tolerate the uncertainty of the situation (Dugas and Robichaud, 2007). Worry can be seen as a coping response that is used to avoid the distress associated with uncertainty. Experimental manipulations of intolerance of uncertainty show a direct relationship between uncertainty and level of worrying (Ladouceur et al, 2000). Intolerance of uncertainty is also correlated with difficulty in tolerating distressing experiences (Lee et al, 2010).

The idea that worry is a coping response that has an avoidant function was first introduced by Borkovec (1994). The verbal act of worrying is experienced as aversive, but it may paradoxically be keeping more unpleasant experiences, which are often imagery based, at bay. For a man with oesophageal cancer, worrying about what might happen to him and how he is going to cope may be less distressing than facing the images of dying from a haematemesis that are at the back of his mind.

This research has informed the treatment of worry in patients with generalized anxiety disorder (Wells, 2000; Dugas and Robichaud, 2007), and can guide us in work on worry with people who have cancer. Montel (2010) has provided a description of a case report of the treatment of generalized anxiety in a woman with breast cancer.

Working with beliefs about worry

Cognitive techniques can be used to identify and test beliefs about worry, and these can lead on to behavioural experiments. For instance, a belief that there is nothing you can do to cope with worry might be tested by scheduling 'worry time' for half an hour a day. When a worry comes up, patients put it aside until their 'appointment' with themselves. Many people find that by the time the appointment comes up, the worry is no longer so dominant. Beliefs about the need always to think the worst and not tempt fate can initially be tested in relation to worries about everyday things. For a few days the patient can be asked to make negative predictions as usual about their life, and then to assume the best. They can then record what the actual outcome was, and they will soon realize that there is no relationship between their predictions and what actually happens. They can then practise generating positive outcomes rather than their habitual negative outcomes.

Moving from worry to problem solving

Teaching the patient basic problem-solving techniques can be very effective in managing worry. Many people find the use of a 'worry tree' helpful (see Figure 10.2). Differentiating between problems over which the patient can exert some control (which require skilful problem solving) and problems that

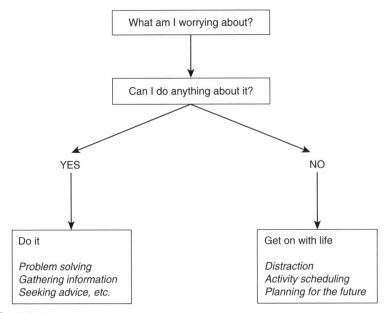

Fig. 10.2 'Worry tree.'

they cannot control (which necessitate a letting go) can sometimes break into the worry cycle.

Tolerating uncertainty

The whole experience of having cancer is one of uncertainty. If a patient has an 80% chance of 5-year survival, they cannot be certain that they will not be among the 20% of patients who die. If a person has an incurable condition, they know that they will die but they cannot know when. Therefore it is not surprising that people who already have difficulty living with uncertainty in their life develop an anxious preoccupation when they have cancer. Experiments can be set up to test the belief that not knowing or not being in control is intolerable. These are usually best done with everyday activities outside the cancer situation (e.g. a patient who is constantly seeking reassurance from their partner can start by making small decisions about what to have for dinner). The patient should expect to feel anxious and uncomfortable while doing these experiments. The aim is not to cope perfectly without any distress, but rather, as Gil Fronsdal says, to be a little more 'comfortable with being uncomfortable.' Mindfulness practice (see Chapter 7) may help to allowing the patient to live with uncertainty without reacting.

Overcoming cognitive avoidance

Dugas and Robichaud (2007) have a module in their treatment for generalized anxiety disorder that involves exposure in imagination to one's worst hypothetical fears. This is a form of decatastrophizing. Many of the deepest fears of people with cancer are not directly related to the threat of death, and these may well be amenable to this intervention. For instance, a 30-year-old woman who had recently completed treatment for breast cancer was confident that she could beat the disease. However, when she met a potential new partner she became preoccupied with the notion that, even though she had told him about her illness and he had been very accepting, he would leave her. She ruminated about this constantly, mentally rerunning their conversations for signs of rejection, and she constantly sought reassurance about their meaning from her friends. The therapist asked her to imagine the worst-case scenario – her new partner telling her that he did not want to see her any more – and to allow herself to stay with the image, the emotional impact, and the unpleasant body sensations without thinking about ways to reassure herself. She felt nauseous when she did this, but was surprised to find that she was able to tolerate the sensations. By practising this when her fears arose she found that the aversive experience became more bearable. She did some problem solving about what she would do if the relationship ended, and found that she had broken the worry cycle.

Again, mindfulness practice (see Chapter 7) may be used to help the patient to stay with their unpleasant experiences, following the ebb and flow of feelings, and noticing how the distress does not remain constant but changes and, with time, dissipates.

Dugas and Robichaud (2007) advise that if fear of relapse is the central theme of worry, it may still be possible to use this technique so long as the risk of relapse is not high and the patient is willing to undergo the exposure task. In other circumstances they suggest using problem-solving or emotional regulation strategies.

Panic

We have encountered vicious circles of anxiety throughout this chapter. In some circumstances these can become a spiral of increasing anxiety that culminates in a panic attack. Anxiety is associated with a range of physiological symptoms, such as palpitations, breathlessness, sweating, light-headedness and shaking. If these are interpreted as signs of an impending catastrophe, the patient will become increasingly anxious. There is a direct link between the physiological sensation and the catastrophic thought:

Palpitations: 'I'm going to have a heart attack.'

Breathlessness: 'I'm going to suffocate.'

Dizziness: 'I'm going to collapse.'

Not surprisingly, we take evasive action on the basis of our catastrophic thought, so if we believe that we are suffocating we open the window to get more air, or if we fear that we will collapse we hold on to something. These safety behaviours further reinforce the belief by appearing to confirm that if we had not taken this action the consequence would have been terrible. Once we have experienced panic attacks we may start to avoid situations that we find uncomfortable or where we would not be able to access help.

Treatment for panic involves exploring collaboratively the patient's physical sensations, thoughts, emotions, and behaviours, together with the context or situation in which they occurred. This should be done sensitively, as people with serious physical illness may resent being told that their thoughts about their physical sensations are 'distorted' (for a description of the use of Socratic questioning in people facing adversity, see Moorey, 2011). The patient then monitors the panic attacks and together with the therapist starts to explore the alternative explanation for the attacks. The most important part of the therapy is devising experiments to test the new, less catastrophic explanation by dropping safety behaviours and overcoming avoidance (Bennett-Levy et al, 2004). For example, Fred, a 70-year-old man with progressive lung cancer, found that he became breathless on exertion and would have panic attacks because he feared 'this was the time' that he was going to die, because he would stop breathing. The therapist identified two safety behaviours:

1. rushing to get across the bathroom to get his morning ablutions over as quickly as possible
2. breathing more quickly to take in more air.

The simple experiment consisted of taking his time in the bathroom and learning some controlled breathing techniques so that he slowed down his breathing and stopped hyperventilating. He found that he actually felt less breathless when he tried the alternative strategy, and his panic and anxiety decreased.

In most cases, panic can be treated in the same way as it would be in people without physical illness. However, certain behavioural experiments should be used with caution in patients with active or advanced disease. Patients with lung disease should not be asked to do hyperventilation experiments to demonstrate the effect of overbreathing on panic symptoms (in Fred's case it was sufficient to teach him a controlled breathing technique to stop the hyperventilation), and patients with advanced disease may not be able to use more active experiments (e.g. running up stairs to increase their heart rate).

Cognitive interventions for helpless/hopeless patients

For the helpless/hopeless patient, cancer represents loss, and the future is perceived as a bleak certainty. Whereas the anxious patient feels out of control but tries to remain in control, the helpless/hopeless patient, believing the situation to be essentially uncontrollable, has given up. This model can inform the cognitive techniques that are chosen. The methods that are used challenge the pessimistic certainty that the future is hopeless. They also help to give the patient a sense of personal control. The therapist and the patient work collaboratively to establish from the information available how bleak the future really is. Evidence for the patient's belief that the future is hopeless is examined, and evidence against this belief is weighed up. In situations where there is a good chance of recovery this involves testing unrealistic pessimism. However, hope for the future does not rest solely on evidence that there is a chance of a cure. *A positive approach to the rest of one's life, no matter how short that may be, can contribute to quality of life.* In patients with a poorer prognosis, hope may be about finding things to look forward to on a day-to-day basis. Identifying the specific negative belief is very important here, because it is easy to make assumptions about what the patient is thinking in an emotionally charged situation. The therapist may think 'If I was in this situation I would feel this way', but their assumptions about what the patient is thinking may be based more on their own reactions than on the patient's view of his or her illness (Moorey, 2011).

Many patients think that if they cannot do all that they used to be able to do, it's not worth doing anything at all. Demonstrating this all-or-nothing thinking is one strategy that can be used with a helpless/hopeless patient. The helpless patient is usually seeing the options in a dichotomous way, as if they can either be in total control of the situation or they are completely helpless. Since so much of the fight against cancer is out of their control, they are in a helpless role. The therapist needs to show the patient that with a disease like cancer we can only really work with probabilities, not certainties. In fact this is not any different from any other risk in life. For example, never smoking a cigarette decreases your risk of getting lung cancer, but does not reduce it to zero, and wearing a seatbelt means that you are less likely to be seriously injured in a road traffic accident, but does not guarantee this.

This can be emphasized by asking the patient to rate the degree of control that they have over various occurrences in life, and to compare these with their control over cancer. An analogue scale can be used to demonstrate that control lies along a continuum, from no control at one end to total control at the other:

No control [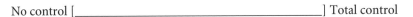] Total control

Searching for alternatives is used to explore activities that the patient can still do despite having cancer. The patient lists all those activities that he or she is still capable of doing. As with all CBT, the patient is encouraged to monitor and challenge automatic thoughts, but not everyone is able to use the daily record of automatic thoughts fluently. Table 10.3 shows the automatic thoughts and alternative responses of a patient with a salivary tumour who was able to make limited use of the method.

Table 10.3 Record of automatic thoughts of a patient with a salivary tumour

Automatic thoughts	Alternative responses
I have cancer – I know I do	The hospital says I have not got cancer
Sometimes I wish this lump in my mouth was cancer so I could get rid of it	You don't because you would not like to go through all that again (i.e. more treatment)
Life is not worth living. I have not changed my life since I've been ill, and the cancer will come back	I've got to go on for my family I can do things to change my life

Another woman with a second recurrence of breast cancer felt very sad and hopeless. During the therapy session she was taught how to record and challenge her thoughts. The thoughts and responses that she produced in the session are shown in Table 10.4.

CBT in action

If we again consider the case of Jenny, described in Chapter 8, we can view cognitive techniques in action. This 45-year-old patient was a divorced teacher with an 8-year-old son. Her response to having breast cancer was to feel depressed, hopeless, and angry. We have seen how activity scheduling and goal planning helped her to feel less hopeless during the first phase of therapy (see p. 116). Cognitive interventions began in the first treatment session, and addressed her hopeless feelings. The therapist elicited automatic thoughts which confirmed that Jenny had a negative view of herself ('I'm useless', 'I'm handicapped') as well as a negative view of the future ('What's the point of doing anything if the cancer might come back?'). She was interpreting cancer as creating a present and permanent loss from her personal domain. She had lost her ability to function as an independent, normal person, and she did not believe that this would ever return. These hopeless thoughts had to be dealt with before the behavioural homework was set. In the next session Jenny was asked to start recording her thoughts, and the concept of reality testing was explained to her. She took well to the task of monitoring and challenging negative automatic thoughts (see Table 10.5).

She was due to receive a course of adjuvant chemotherapy, but was very concerned about the possible side-effects. She described how she felt that just as she was beginning to do more and feel more in control of her life, she would be tired and ill as a result of the treatment. The therapist helped her to test this

Table 10.4 Automatic thoughts of a woman with recurring breast cancer

Situation	Emotions	Automatic thoughts	Alternative response
Enjoying a day in the sun	Sad (80%)	I won't be around to see this sun for much longer (90%)	I will be (50%) The doctor says I'm responding to treatment (90%) I've got to be around to look after the kids (90%) I know of a woman who has had cancer in her breast, spine, and liver for 15 years. If she can do it, I can do it (70%) If I don't enjoy it now it's like giving up (80%)

Table 10.5 Negative automatic thoughts recorded and evaluated by Jenny

Situation	Emotions	Automatic thoughts	Alternative response
Thinking about friends	Alone Depressed	My life has become a nightmare. It's out of my control	If I make a conscious effort I can maintain some control
In the kitchen	Despondent	Once the chemotherapy gets going there are lots of things I won't want to eat and I'll start losing weight again	I can buy convenience foods because it's probably the effort of preparing the foods that's the problem
Working at something	Anxious	I've only got a fraction of the energy I used to have, and that could be permanent	I may be depressed. Even if I feel tired, it's better to stay active because I will achieve more
Getting up in the morning	Sad	There are so many things I haven't done and will never do	People do different things in life, and mine hasn't been so bad. I could make an effort to do what I want to do

automatic thought by questioning her about the evidence that chemotherapy had to be so toxic. In fact she had already had a short course of chemotherapy before starting radiotherapy, and had not felt significantly unwell. The therapist then went on to ask about the advantages and disadvantages to her of receiving treatment. Jenny came up with the following list:

Advantages   *Disadvantages*

I won't have regrets and worries   I will lose weight

I may have a statistical advantage   I will be tired and find
and live longer   everything difficult

I won't be able to talk to people   I will be able to look after my son for sick
without feeling   longer

I will become sterile

This procedure helped to put Jenny's ideas about chemotherapy into perspective. Here is her own account of the cognitive techniques that she learned to use in therapy.

When I stopped having overwhelming negative thoughts but went on monitoring what I was thinking, I was surprised to discover that a great number of my thoughts were negative in one way or another, and that I seem to have a bottomless fund of them. Negative thoughts seemed to hang together like a string of sausages, and I gradually found that it was a good idea to try to snip them off. I understood what the therapist was saying about thoughts containing distortions . . . and I found that sometimes I could deal with my thoughts in a different way, taking account of the fact that they could contain a lot of mistakes, and noticing when a train of thought was leading to no good.

Summary

In this chapter we have looked at how CBT can be applied to two of the commonest emotional reactions in patients with cancer. When the patient's focus is on the threat that cancer poses and their uncertainty about their ability to control the situation, they feel anxious. We have considered some ways of managing anxious preoccupation, how to deal with fear of recurrence, and how to manage worry and panic. When we are overwhelmed by the threat and feel completely unable to impose any control on the situation, we become helpless and hopeless. We have considered some methods for inducing hope, and have presented a case example of CBT in action.

Chapter 11

Applications of cognitive and behavioural techniques to common problems

Cognitive and behavioural techniques for anxiety and depression remain the core of CBT for people with cancer, but they are by no means the only problems which may need to be addressed during therapy. In this chapter we shall consider some common cancer-related problems and discuss the interventions that can be used with them.

We shall consider the following:

◆ working with anger and self-blame

◆ insomnia and fatigue

◆ pain

◆ nausea.

Working with anger and self-blame

Some methods that can be used for ventilating and channelling anger were described in Chapter 7. Here we shall present some of the more cognitive and behavioural methods for managing anger. More information on cognitive behavioural methods for managing anger can be found in Burns (1980), Novaco (1976, 1995), Novaco and Chemtob (1998), and Deffenbacher (1999). The literature on anger management in cancer patients is still sparse, but meta-analyses have found moderate effects of anger management interventions based on CBT (Beck and Fernandez, 1998; DiGiuseppe and Tafrate, 2003). Figure 11.1 outlines a simple model of the processes that occur in people with anger problems. The patient with cancer will come to a situation primed with schemas that may make him or her prone to view the situation as an attack or violation. The situation may be directly connected with cancer, and so the unfairness of the person's position is highlighted ('This shouldn't be happening to me'). On other occasions, the trigger may be unrelated to cancer, but because the sense of injustice is present in the person's mind, they are primed

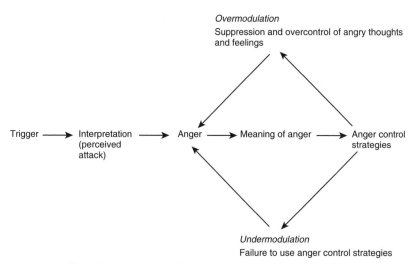

Overmodulation
Suppression and overcontrol of angry thoughts
and feelings

Trigger ⟶ Interpretation ⟶ Anger ⟶ Meaning of anger ⟶ Anger control
              (perceived   strategies
              attack)

Undermodulation
Failure to use anger control strategies

Fig. 11.1 Outline of the sequence of events in anger problems.

to find injustice in the way they are being treated. Thus the underlying resentment of the disease leads to a misinterpretation of events as unfair. Sometimes there may be underlying beliefs about the way people should behave towards a person who is ill ('They should treat me more respectfully'), which activate the anger. Once the situation has been interpreted as an unjust attack or a violation of a rule, the emotion of anger is experienced. The way in which the person views these angry feelings will then determine the consequences. If they view anger as undesirable, dangerous, and something to be avoided, the individual will try to suppress it or over-regulate it. This may lead to breakthrough anger and the other problems associated with emotional suppression that were described in Chapter 7, and requires intervention to facilitate engagement with feelings and their constructive expression. If the anger is perceived as justified, this may mean that the individual does not try to regulate it. This failure of control strategies leads to further anger.

Here we shall consider three basic steps in an anger management programme, namely establishing motivation to change, identifying cues and automatic thoughts, and developing a cognitive behavioural strategy for change.

Establishing motivation to change

It is socially acceptable to think that it is unjust and unfair for a person to have cancer. It can also be quite exhilarating to feel righteous indignation, and this is more empowering than feeling like a helpless victim. When this anger leads the patient to effective problem solving, constructive action to improve services, helping other patients, etc., it is healthy and useful. However, sometimes anger does not lead to behavioural activation, but may paralyse the patient with impotent rage. At this point it is helpful to explore the benefits and costs of continuing to be so angry. The most useful focus is not on the anger that the person feels about the disease, but on the anger that is projected or generalized elsewhere. This is not a primary emotion in the sense of a healthy and appropriate response to the disease, but an inappropriate overgeneralization. Distinguishing between the two allows a therapeutic alliance to be developed with an agreement between the patient and the therapist to work on controlling the maladaptive anger. Guided discovery is used to show the patient how the understandable anger about cancer is spilling over into other areas of life, with undesirable effects. The therapist should acknowledge the benefits of feeling angry (e.g. not feeling helpless, feeling activated, feeling right) before going on to any challenging, because this will increase the patient's motivation to change, and will reduce the possibility of a breakdown in the alliance.

Identifying cues and automatic thoughts

Once the costs of anger have been established (e.g. rows with family members, feeling tense, wasting precious energy), information can be gathered about the triggers for angry outbursts. As with any other problem, the patient is asked to record angry situations and identify cues for anger. Automatic thoughts are elicited as described above. There is often a sequence that leads to angry outbursts (see Figure 11.1), and it is worth going through the sequence in some detail to establish which actions and thoughts were important in producing the final result.

At the first stage of appraisal one cognitive distortion is very common. 'Should' statements appear again and again in people's thought records:

'This shouldn't have happened to me!'
'It's not fair, I've been a good person, I shouldn't be treated this way.'
'He should be much more considerate!'
'He should spend more time with me!'

Although the anger may be directed at God or at fate, excessive anger usually has an impact at an interpersonal level. It is not the railing at fate that causes problems, but the snapping at one's children. In these situations there is usually a sense of some rule being contravened ('They should have known I was tired' or 'They shouldn't make so much noise'). It is vital to gather information about this before moving on to challenging the distorted thinking.

At the next stage, some people may 'overmodulate' their anger and require emotion-based interventions, whereas others may 'undermodulate' their anger.

They may not have strategies that they can use to prevent the escalation of anger, such as standing back from their angry feelings, distracting themselves by counting to 10, taking a deep breath, talking to themselves ('Don't go over the top now – it isn't that important'), and walking away from the situation. People who get angry under stress may not have learned these strategies, or may be so stressed that they are not using them. This phase of analysing the cues for anger and the patient's reaction allows the therapist to ascertain the extent to which the patient uses adaptive or maladaptive coping strategies.

Developing a strategy for change

Once the sequence of actions and thoughts has been established, the therapist can work with the patient to find the weak point in the chain. The cognitive behavioural analysis may reveal a pattern like that shown in Figure 11.2. *Analysis of the cues* for anger can often suggest interventions to reduce the likelihood of anger being provoked. For example, difficult situations can be avoided, or the environment can be changed to reduce the frequency of their occurrence. In the case shown in Figure 11.2, establishing a rule that the children

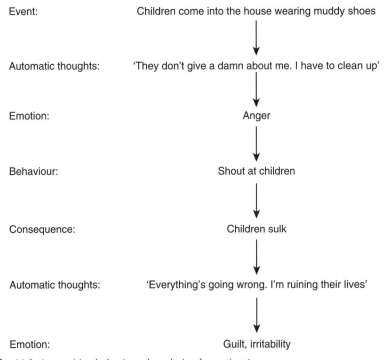

Event:	Children come into the house wearing muddy shoes
Automatic thoughts:	'They don't give a damn about me. I have to clean up'
Emotion:	Anger
Behaviour:	Shout at children
Consequence:	Children sulk
Automatic thoughts:	'Everything's going wrong. I'm ruining their lives'
Emotion:	Guilt, irritability

Fig. 11.2 A cognitive behavioural analysis of a patient's anger.

must change their shoes before coming into the house might help to reduce the likelihood of the patient's anger being triggered.

Identifying and challenging distorted thinking obviously plays an important part in the anger control techniques of APT. When the anger is interpersonally based, techniques to encourage empathy can be particularly important. The patient may be asked to consider the situation from the other person's perspective. If this is ineffective, more active methods such as role playing the other person in the interaction may produce a shift. *Empathy techniques* help to show the patient that the person with whom they are angry is not usually attacking or hurting them deliberately. In the examples cited in Figure 11.2, the patient might respond to her automatic thoughts by saying:

1. 'My children love me, but when they're excited they can't think ahead. There's no reason why they can't help by washing the floor.'

2. 'Only one thing is wrong – the floor is dirty. If I can control my irritability, my children are not going to suffer.'

Once the common thread of 'shoulds' has been identified across angry situations, the patient can monitor their 'shoulds' and replace them with more adaptive interpretations. Following on from this, the therapist can look at the advantages and disadvantages of working from a 'should'-based belief system, and examine the evidence that the world really works according to the rules that the patient applies.

Once anger has been activated, the patient has a choice of several different coping strategies *to reduce their affect* (e.g. calming self-instructions such as 'It's all right, I can handle this without blowing my top', distraction, or relaxation). The therapist and the patient may need to work on how the patient can respond assertively without getting angry, and this may require role play during the session. The patient can rehearse in role play how to show appropriate anger and achieve their goal. Unassertive people sometimes alternate between being passive doormats and exploding with anger. Patients who suppress their anger often fear that when they change they will become 'nasty' people or lose control. Cognitive techniques can be used to test these beliefs, and behavioural experiments can be set up to find out whether saying no or standing up for yourself really does lead to the dire consequences predicted by the unassertive person. The therapist helps the patient to distinguish between appropriate and useful emotions and behaviours (healthy, constructive anger and assertion) and maladaptive ones (impotent rage and aggressiveness) (see Box 11.1).

Insomnia

Insomnia is a common problem in people with cancer, with up to 40% of patients reporting poor sleep (Savard and Morin, 2001; Savard et al, 2001;

Box 11.1 Methods for dealing with anger about cancer

In the following example, the patient had expressed their anger as follows:
'I've lived a good life. Why should I get this when bad people go scot-free?'

1. Encourage direct expression of this anger in the session and to significant others.

2. Find appropriate outlets for the angry feelings.

3. Reality-test the belief that life should be fair.

   (a) Assess the evidence that life is fair.

   (b) Consider people whom the patient has known who have had cancer. How many of them were good and how many were bad?

4. Look for alternative ways of viewing the situation. For example, one patient felt better when she stopped asking 'Why me?' and started asking 'Why not me?'

5. Identify the cognitive distortion (the tyranny of the 'shoulds').

6. Find the origin of the belief (e.g. in childhood experience or religion) so that it can be reframed as a learned rule rather than a universal fact.

Davidson et al, 2002). It is linked to both fatigue (Zee and Ancoli-Israel, 2009) and worry. Poor sleep may well be a problem that people undergoing a course of APT want to address, and sleep difficulties can be incorporated into the overall conceptualization quite easily. As always, developing a formulation of the factors that are maintaining the problem is the key to understanding and treating the condition. Identifying the physical factors that are affecting sleep should of course be the priority. Pain and breathlessness are probably the most common of these, and are seen in patients with more advanced disease. The therapist should liaise with the primary care or palliative care team to make sure that these symptoms are investigated fully, that adequate pain control is established, and that management of any respiratory condition is optimized. Once this has been done, CBT for insomnia utilizes a range of techniques that address both behavioural factors (environmental context, sleep habits, and unhelpful use of alcohol and sedatives) and cognitive factors (dysfunctional beliefs about sleep, and worry). It usually combines advice on sleep hygiene with changing sleep-related behaviours and evaluating unhelpful thinking (Smith and Neubauer, 2003). Improvement in sleep following CBT appears to be associated with changes in dysfunctional beliefs about sleep and a reduction in daytime naps (Tremblay et al, 2009).

Self-monitoring and sleep hygiene

The first step is to ask the patient to keep a sleep diary. This can monitor several different variables, but will usually include the time they went to bed, how long it took them to fall asleep, how many times they woke during the night, when they got up, and their automatic thoughts. Sleep hygiene instructions usually consist of advice about what to do in the evening to reduce insomnia, and instructions about sleep and the bedroom environment.

Evening routine

- Avoid caffeine, alcohol, and smoking in the evening.
- Avoid drinking too much liquid in the evening.
- Eat regular meals and do not go to bed hungry.
- Exercise regularly during the day, but not within 3 hours of bedtime.
- Develop a bedtime routine in which you wind down by making a hot drink, reading, etc.

Sleep

- Get up at the same time each day.
- Sleep only as much as you need to in order to feel refreshed during the day; don't spend longer in bed to try to catch up on sleep.
- Avoid taking naps during the day.
- Don't try to fall asleep.

Bedroom

- Eliminate disturbing light or noise.
- Avoid any activities other than sleep and sex (do not have a TV in the bedroom).

Stimulus control

This is a well-established technique based on the principle that in insomnia the individual's bed becomes associated with being awake and ruminating. The idea is to break this conditioning and associate bed with sleep. The patient is asked to get up at the same time each day, to restrict sleep to the bedroom, and to use the bedroom only for sleeping and sex. To break the cycle of waking and spending time in bed worrying about cancer or insomnia, the patient is asked to get out of bed if they are awake for more than 15–20 minutes. They should only return to bed when they feel sleepy.

Relaxation

Relaxation techniques such as those described in Chapter 8 can also be very helpful.

Cognitive techniques

Worry about recurrence or disease progression is a very common feature of insomnia in patients with cancer. This can contribute to difficulty in getting off to sleep and difficulty in returning to sleep when they have woken during the night. The sleep hygiene and stimulus control interventions can help to prevent the person's bed becoming associated with worry. Another tip is to keep a notepad by the bedside. When a thought comes up, the patient can jot it down. This act of externalizing the worry sometimes allows the patient to let go. The techniques described in Chapter 10 can be applied equally effectively to daytime or night-time worry.

In addition to this primary worry about cancer, patients may also worry about the insomnia itself. They may catastrophize about the effect of a sleepless night on their performance the next day, or worry that the lack of sleep might make their cancer worse. Reality testing can be used to assess the likelihood of these feared consequences, and behavioural experiments can be used to test the beliefs. For instance, a patient's fear that they will feel terrible the next day or that they won't be able to concentrate can be tested by asking them to keep a diary of their sleep and their performance.

Fatigue

Fatigue is the most frequently reported symptom associated with cancer and its treatment (Hofmana et al, 2007). Not surprisingly, there is a strong association between insomnia and fatigue in people with cancer (Zee et al, 2009), and cognitive behavioural interventions for fatigue will often need to incorporate work on insomnia as well (Armes et al, 2007). A good maintenance conceptualization is needed to guide treatment. The activity schedule can be adapted to record activity and fatigue, and thoughts about tiredness can be monitored. This will give information about the vicious circles of negative thinking, avoidance, and fatigue that can occur in people with cancer. For example, Frank was a 79-year-old man with metastatic prostate cancer. He felt tired all the time and found it painful to exert himself too much. The activity schedule revealed that he spent a lot of time lying on the sofa watching TV. During these periods he rated his fatigue level as high. He was surprised to discover that he became slightly less fatigued when he was up doing things. The thought record contained many automatic thoughts about his disease, his tiredness, and his pain, and the therapist was able to elicit a belief that 'If I overdo it I might make everything worse.' Some discussion and reality testing established that activity would not make his cancer worse, and Frank could see that his inactivity was leading to more worry, and was possibly making him even more tired. He decided to experiment with spending less time on the sofa, and made sure that he walked round to the shop to buy a paper every day. He discovered that his pain did not get any worse when he was more active, and his tiredness actually decreased.

Interventions for fatigue involve identifying negative beliefs about exercise, and then testing them through guided discovery and behavioural experiments. Such experiments will usually involve the use of an activity schedule to monitor symptoms and a graded task assignment to gradually increase the patient's exercise levels.

Pain

One-third of people with cancer experience pain, and this figure rises to 75% in patients with advanced cancer. Up to 50% of cancer patients do not feel that they have adequate pain control (Larue et al, 1995; Zech et al, 1995) There is strong evidence for the effectiveness of CBT in cancer pain management (see Chapter 3). As with fatigue and insomnia, the beliefs that patients have about their pain will influence their coping behaviours. Catastrophic fears about the meaning of pain and beliefs about the control of pain are the two main themes that seem to be present in people who experience significant distress with pain, even when receiving appropriate analgesia. Catastrophic interpretations of pain also fall into two categories, namely fears that the pain is an indication of disease spread, and fears that it is a sign that the patient's behaviour is in some way making things worse. Automatic thoughts such as 'I'm sure this shouldn't hurt like this – there must be something wrong' contribute to an anxious preoccupation, with the consequent worry, reassurance seeking, and checking that are seen with this adjustment style. Automatic thoughts such as 'I'd better not exert myself in case it makes this worse' lead to guarding and avoidance of activity. Both of these catastrophic thinking styles will be associated with monitoring of body sensations and increased attention to painful stimuli. Figure 11.3 shows a visual representation of the interactions between thoughts, anxiety, and behaviour in pain.

Working with these cognitions involves psychoeducation about the nature of pain, reality testing, and then setting up experiments to test what happens if the patient changes the focus of attention, checks less often, and seeks less reassurance.

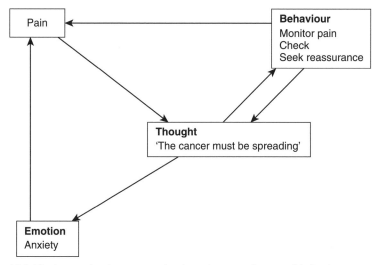

Fig. 11.3 The interaction between pain, thoughts, emotions, and behaviour.

The degree to which an individual feels that they have control over their pain also influences the experience of pain, and people who feel that they cannot control their pain will feel helpless and hopeless. There are several techniques that have been shown to be effective in managing pain, and these will be particularly helpful for patients who have such beliefs. Keeping a pain diary can begin to delineate situations or activities that relieve or exacerbate symptoms. Setting appropriate goals and adopting a graded approach can build a sense of self-efficacy. Patients who are not aware of the factors that might influence their pain can become caught in a vicious circle of underactivity when the pain is worse, and overactivity when the pain is reduced. Pacing activities can be helpful. Specific pain management strategies such as distraction and relaxation techniques may also be useful.

Nausea

Nausea is a debilitating side-effect of chemotherapy, although as a result of reductions in the toxicity of chemotherapy regimes and improvements in anti-emetic drugs its prevalence has decreased. Anticipatory nausea is a particularly unpleasant symptom, in which the patient becomes nauseous in anticipation of the chemotherapy treatment. In the past this side-effect developed in 25% of patients by the fourth treatment cycle, but with modern treatments fewer than 10% of patients display symptoms of anticipatory nausea per treatment cycle, and 2% or fewer have symptoms of anticipatory vomiting

(Aapro et al, 2005). Anticipatory nausea is associated with the number of treatment cycles and with poorer control of nausea during treatment, so there is strong evidence for an underlying classical conditioning effect. However, levels of anxiety, expectations of being nauseous (Montgomery and Bovbjerg, 2001), and family support (Kim and Morrow, 2007) are other factors that are implicated in its genesis.

Factors that predict anticipatory nausea (Morrow, 1984; Morrow et al, 1991) include the following:

1. age < 50 years
2. nausea and vomiting after the last chemotherapy
3. describing nausea after the last treatment as 'moderate, severe, or intolerable'
4. reporting the side-effect 'warm or hot all over' after the last treatment
5. susceptibility to motion sickness
6. experiencing 'sweating' after the last treatment
7. experiencing 'generalized weakness' after the last treatment.

Whereas 5-hydroxytryptamine type 3 receptor antagonists provide relief for chemotherapy-induced nausea and vomiting, they do not appear to control anticipatory nausea and vomiting (Figueroa-Moseley et al, 2007). The Antiemetic Subcommittee of the Multinational Association of Supportive Care in Cancer (MASCC) stated in 1998 that 'the best treatment for anticipatory emesis is the best possible control of acute and delayed emesis', and subsequently added that benzodiazepines and behavioural interventions represented the best evidence for treatment of this condition (Aapro et al, 2005).

The behavioural interventions for the treatment of anticipatory nausea and vomiting are based on the principles of exposure. The patient is exposed to stimuli that trigger nausea either in their imagination or *in vivo* for sufficient time for their nausea to decrease, and with repeated exposure this leads to a reduction in the severity of symptoms.

Identify stimuli that trigger nausea

The commonest stimuli are olfactory (e.g. smell of the hospital, smell of the hospital café) and cognitive (e.g. thinking about going to the hospital), but other stimuli (e.g. travelling on the bus to the appointment) and mood state can also trigger nausea (Fernandez-Marcos et al, 1996). A hierarchy is constructed, with the stimuli that produce least nausea and anxiety at the top (an example is shown in Table 11.1). It is important to ensure that the intervals between the items in the hierarchy are fairly even, because if the patient has to

Table 11.1 Hierarchy of stimuli that produce nausea

Trigger	Level of nausea (on a scale of 0–100)
Smell of any food	10
Being driven in the car	15
Driving past the hospital	25
Imagining the chemotherapy treatment	60
Smell of the hospital	80
Chemotherapy room	100

suddenly move up from a low level to a high one this may make the task too difficult.

Exposure to stimuli

The patient starts at the bottom of the hierarchy and arranges exposure to the situation or trigger. The instructions are to stay in the situation for long enough to allow the nausea to decrease to a manageable level. It is not essential to remain until the nausea has disappeared completely. This is repeated until the situation does not trigger significant nausea, and then the patient moves to the next item in the hierarchy. Exposure is more effective if it is undertaken using the real stimulus rather than in imagination, and if it is prolonged and repeated. It may be helpful for the therapist to assist the patient in some of these sessions, but this is not essential, and self-guided exposure is very cost-effective. Relaxation may be helpful in allowing the patient to stay with the nausea during exposure, but should be used with care in case it becomes a safety behaviour.

With the hierarchy presented here the therapist might initially demonstrate that the patient can tolerate smells by bringing food into the session and asking the patient to sit with it in the room. The patient is asked to rate their level of distress or nausea on a scale of 0–100 at periodic intervals, and the reduction in level can be plotted on a graph. Following this the patient could practise exposure at home, starting with food that they can tolerate, and moving up to more nausea-inducing smells.

The next step in the hierarchy, being driven in the car, might be something that the patient can do with a family member as a self-help assignment. Again the principle of beginning with a manageable task (e.g. driving close to home) and then progressing to more difficult ones (e.g. driving closer to the hospital, past familiar landmarks and road signs associated with going for treatment) is applied, so that each exercise can become a success experience.

The cognitive stimulus of imagining the chemotherapy treatment can be addressed in two ways:

1. through exposure in imagination, where the patient creates an image of the chemotherapy room or talks through the steps in the treatment

2. by unpacking some of the elements of the imagery and carrying out *in-vivo* exposure (e.g. looking at pictures of hospital interiors, holding a syringe and drip apparatus).

This will lead on to the item at the top of the hierarchy, which involves being in the hospital chemotherapy room. This may need to be a therapist-aided session with the patient gradually moving through the hospital, waiting at each stage until distress levels become manageable, and then moving on further until they get to the chemotherapy room. In these exercises it is helpful to have the hospital staff on board with the procedure. They will then be able to provide equipment for exposure sessions and access to chemotherapy areas.

Cognitive techniques

So far we have described the procedure in purely behavioural terms, but exposure can be enhanced when it is embedded within a cognitive behavioural conceptualization. Patients have expectations and beliefs about chemotherapy that may be distorted or unhelpful. For example:

'It's inevitable that I'm going to be sick'
'I won't be able to stand it'
'I can't cope'
'If I vomit everyone will stare at me'
'I won't be able to stand the embarrassment.'

These thoughts can be evaluated using the techniques described in Chapters 9 and 10. Verbal discussion will help to reduce these beliefs to some extent, but its main role is to help to motivate the patient to engage in behavioural experiments. The exposure tasks can be targeted to test specific beliefs, and this can accelerate the process.

For instance, a patient who believed that she could never cope with nausea and could not see how anyone could tolerate feeling sick was shown a video of someone describing their experience of chemotherapy. The therapist then took the patient to the hospital and stood with her in the foyer while they tested the belief that she would not be able to stay for more than 2 minutes. She tolerated 5 minutes, and then with support from the therapist extended this to 10 minutes, thus disconfirming her prediction.

Using this model of targeting exposure to test specific beliefs, it may be possible to carry out the treatment in a single extended session over a period of

2 to 3 hours. Single-session exposure has been evaluated in individuals with simple phobias, but to our knowledge has not been researched in the treatment of anticipatory nausea and vomiting.

Coping with chemotherapy

A range of coping strategies are available to help people to cope with the treatment session itself. These include relaxation and distraction methods, such as listening to an MP3 player or playing computer games.

Summary

CBT is not limited to the treatment of anxiety and depression. It can help patients to cope with other emotions, such as anger, and has a place in the management of some of the symptoms that are commonly encountered in cancer. This chapter has described how the therapy can be adapted for the treatment of cancer-related insomnia, fatigue, pain, and nausea. The same basic techniques can be used in all of these areas, but the model is refined for each problem so that cognitive and behavioural interventions, especially behavioural experiments, can be targeted more effectively.

Chapter 12

Cancer in context: Working with underlying beliefs and assumptions

One of the strengths of CBT is its flexibility in providing a formulation of problems both at a cross-sectional or maintenance level (the here and now) and at a deeper developmental or longitudinal level. Although most of our short-term problem-focused work with patients is in the here and now, it is sometimes helpful to understand the problems in more historical terms. In this chapter we shall:

- expand on the developmental model of adjustment to cancer
- explain how to co-create a developmental conceptualization
- describe how cancer has an effect on four different types of belief structures
- outline some methods for working with beliefs.

Personal beliefs and adjustment in cancer

Although intellectually we may recognize that we, like every human being who has ever lived, are going to die, at an emotional level this idea is very difficult to accept. We often act as if we are going to live for ever, and that bad things will somehow not happen to us. Cancer challenges these implicit beliefs about invulnerability and immortality (Janoff-Bullman, 1992). It may also challenge our beliefs that we are competent and able to cope, and that the world is a predictable, fair, and controllable place. As we discussed in Chapter 2, the meaning that patients give to their experience of cancer will depend on their underlying system of beliefs about themselves, other people, and the world around them, as well as on more specific beliefs about illness and its treatment. At the deepest level these beliefs are unconditional, axiomatic assumptions about how things are, and for this reason they have been termed 'core beliefs' (Beck, 1995). They guide us in our general orientation to the world, and if we have had a reasonably supportive and loving upbringing we tend to believe that we are worthwhile, that others are well intentioned, and that the world is a safe place. Cancer challenges these positive beliefs, and patients will feel vulnerable, unable to cope, and hopeless, but in most cases such feelings are only temporary, because the patient is able to find strength and resources to deal with the stress. It may be that most people adapt by integrating the news of their diagnosis into their pre-existing belief system, finding ways to re-establish their sense of being a valued person who has control over a predictable and meaningful environment, and a future that is hopeful. There is some evidence that cancer patients may in fact be more optimistic than healthy controls (Stiegelis et al, 2003).

Positive and negative core beliefs

Most of us tend to have a mixture of positive and negative beliefs, and when we are not under stress the positive beliefs are usually more to the fore. For some people, these positive beliefs are very rigid, perhaps because they have never experienced serious adversity or because they have learned to see things in very black-and-white terms. Their brittle positive core beliefs may be shattered by the trauma of a diagnosis of a terminal illness. It may be that the patient cannot conceptualize what adversity might look like, or it may be that they have very strict ideas about how the world should be. Beliefs that the world is just and predictable make it hard for some people to accommodate their beliefs in the face of trauma (Janoff-Bullman, 1992). They may have assumptions that if they live a good life, or follow certain religious rules, bad things will not happen to them.

For others, a life-threatening illness will confirm some of their secret fears and so activate core beliefs that have been at the back of their mind (e.g. 'I am vulnerable', 'The world is dangerous, unpredictable, and hostile', 'Other people are abusive and unavailable'). These negative core beliefs or schemas often develop as very understandable ways of responding to childhood adversity. If a child is constantly berated for any mistakes that they make, it is reasonable for them to conclude that others will be critical and that perhaps they are in some way inadequate. If their mother who is bringing them up alone is frequently taken into hospital with episodes of depression, the child may decide that people they love will not be there for them, and that they are in some way responsible for this.

Conditional beliefs and compensatory strategies

People who have experienced negative events during their childhood find ways of coping that may be very adaptive at the time, but which may be less helpful in adult life. These 'compensatory strategies' are associated with conditional beliefs that mitigate the unconditional negative beliefs. For instance, the person whose mother suffered bouts of depression might learn that 'If I rely on people I will be let down', and so might construct a self-reliant mode of coping. The person who was constantly being criticized might develop the belief that 'If I get it absolutely right I won't be told off', and so become perfectionistic. These strategies may actually work quite well in adult life – being self-reliant keeps one safe, and being perfectionistic leads to achievement.

However, a diagnosis of a life-threatening illness undermines these well-trodden safety behaviours. When a person has cancer they have to rely on other people, even if it is only the professionals who are treating them. If they are a perfectionist, they will want to know everything about their treatment and try to make sure that they follow it to the letter. The natural tendency will be to use the same strategies that have worked in the past, but these may not be so effective. For instance, a person who experienced significant separations or abuse during their childhood may have core beliefs that the world is a dangerous and unpredictable place in which they are helpless and vulnerable, and where no one can be trusted. To cope with this they may have developed such beliefs as 'If I get close to people they will hurt me' and 'If I can control my life, I will be safe', and used compensatory strategies of avoidance of close relationships, vigilance in avoiding hurt by others, and overcontrol. If they receive a diagnosis of cancer, their fears that the world is dangerous and unpredictable may be confirmed, as will be their sense of vulnerability, but there may be more limited scope to exert their usually controlling strategies. Moreover, they will be forced to become dependent on others for their treatment and care. Therefore their negative beliefs about being harmed and out of control may be activated along with feelings of anxiety and depression.

Core beliefs and personality disorder

Fortunately most of us have positive beliefs and resources, and the compensatory strategies that we use, although not ideal, work for a fair part of the time. Thus although perfectionism, control, dependence on others, self-reliance, etc. may be limiting to some degree, we can still get on with our life. It is only when a major stress such as cancer comes along that we find these strategies wanting. People who have experienced severe disruption to their normal upbringing will have very well-elaborated negative belief systems, but rather impoverished positive beliefs and effective coping strategies. For these people their negative core beliefs are present for much of the time, and having a life-threatening illness simply confirms all of their views. They may have poor problem-solving skills and find themselves in difficult or abusive relationships, or unable to hold down a job, and they may suffer from social isolation. Cancer can then seem like the last straw.

These pervasive negative core beliefs about the self, the world, and other people are usually associated with a diagnosis of personality disorder. People with borderline personality disorder have usually experienced emotional, physical, or sexual abuse in childhood, and will have beliefs that they are bad and incompetent, and that others will be abusive towards or abandon them. Some examples of automatic thoughts arising from these beliefs include the following:

'I deserved to get cancer'
'This is a punishment'
'I can't cope'
'People will take advantage of me'
'It's not fair – bad things always happen to me'
'People will reject me because of my cancer'
'I've got no one to help me.'

Because they move between opposing schemas, they experience rapid changes of emotional state and interpersonal behaviour, shifting from vulnerable help seeking to angry rejection in the space of a single consultation. The compensatory strategies that they use will often be maladaptive (e.g. cutting people out of their lives if they are hurt by them, engaging in self-harm, etc.). When oncology professionals encounter someone with a borderline personality disorder, they can find these reactions very confusing.

Beliefs about illness and adversity

As well as these more general beliefs, attitudes towards health and illness will also influence the meaning that cancer has for each person, and these usually spring from personal experience or things that the patient has heard about cancer. For instance, a woman who has seen a friend lose her hair and become very sick as a result of chemotherapy will be likely to fear the same consequences for herself. The interaction between personal beliefs and beliefs about illness is very important in this context (Williams, 1997). The commonly held belief that cancer means death is an example of this. Other components of the survival schema may also be associated with underlying assumptions. Some of our patients who have experienced several stressful life events over the years, especially if they have a recurrence of the disease, describe a belief that 'they just can't win.' For example, a 40-year-old divorced woman was faced with a recurrence of local breast cancer. Her father had died from carcinoma of the liver in 1978, her mother died from carcinoma of the breast in 1979, and her sister died at the age of 15 years in a road traffic accident. Over the years she had developed the belief that every time she felt life was worth living, something terrible would happen. She had an underlying assumption that 'If I get too cocky, I will be punished for it.' This interfered with her therapy, because every time she thought about trying pleasant activities or doing something to cheer herself up, she also had the thought that something would go wrong. The therapist had to challenge this fatalistic attitude before the patient could continue with therapy. This is an example of a long-standing belief about personal inability to control events, and it is no surprise that this woman developed a helpless/hopeless response to cancer.

The interaction between cancer, other life events, and self-esteem may be a complex one. A middle-aged man had had to cope with a serious injury to his wife, and then himself developed cancer of the mouth. It was only when he was made redundant from work that he became depressed. In this case the cumulative stress, together with the special meaning of loss of livelihood, constituted the threat to his self-esteem.

Developmental conceptualization

The emotional problems that are encountered in oncology are usually less severe and less chronic than those which are found in general psychiatric practice. APT is carried out over 5 to 12 sessions with the majority of patients. Therapy cannot afford to spend too much time on past experiences or seek to change fundamental aspects of personality. The cognitive techniques that have been described in previous chapters are essentially methods of coping which the patient learns during therapy, and then applies after therapy has ended. Problem-solving strategies, planning of time, and evaluation of negative thoughts can all be used to cope with other life stresses in the future. However, within this short-term framework a developmental conceptualization can still prove helpful in guiding therapy, even if core beliefs and conditional beliefs are not directly targeted. For instance, knowing that a patient lost a parent in childhood can alert you to the possibility that beliefs about abandonment and attachment might be important to her, and so help to predict the patient's reactions to therapy. Understanding that witnessing an alcoholic parent has made a person determined never to lose control can help to make sense of their attempts to have total control over their cancer. Sharing this conceptualization with the patient can be very useful. An understanding of the patient's life history and their central beliefs can also make sense of what might seem to be inappropriate coping behaviours. This compassionate, comprehensive conceptualization can help to put the confusing experiences of negative adjustment reactions into context for both the patient and the therapist.

How to co-create a developmental conceptualization

As with all techniques in cognitive therapy, this is most effective if it is done in partnership with the patient. There are no hard-and-fast rules about how this should be done, but a good place to start is generally with the patient's account of how they learned of their diagnosis of cancer.

◆ Did they notice symptoms? What was their initial reaction? How did they deal with it? Did they tell anyone? How long was it before they sought help?

◆ Were they taken seriously at their initial consultation? How did the doctor treat them?

◆ How were they given the bad news? How did they react?

◆ What was the course of their cancer treatment? How did they cope with this? Were their family and friends supportive?

The themes that emerge may be related to real problems in their experience, but they may also give an indication of core beliefs (e.g. feeling completely unsupported, not feeling heard, feeling abused). As we have already discussed, telling their story can be therapeutic in its own right and can aid emotional processing. To set the patient's reaction in context, it is helpful to next ask about their family and personal history.

Family history

1. Parents, brothers and sisters, and extended family.

2. What is the family history of cancer and illness? What are the family's attitudes to cancer and illness?

3. How would the patient describe their parents (e.g. 'Can you describe your mother/father in five words?').

Personal history

1. Early childhood.

2. Any separations, illnesses, hospitalizations, etc.

3. Pre-school relationships with parents, grandparents, and siblings.

4. Schooling (friends, bullying, school refusal, academic achievement).

5. Relationships with family during primary and secondary schooling and adolescence.

6. Occupational history:
   • brief account of jobs held and their duration
   • relationships with work colleagues.

7. Psychosexual history

- How many significant relationships has the patient had? How long did they last?
- Is the patient currently in a relationship? What is the nature of the relationship (e.g. 'Could you describe your partner?')?
- If this has not been covered already, ask how cancer has affected the relationship. Are there more arguments? Is the partner distant or overprotective? Are the patient and their partner talking about the future?

General coping style

1. Check for any other stressful life events in the past.
2. How does the patient usually cope with stress?
3. What does the patient think others would say are his or her strengths?
4. Is the patient calling on these strengths now? If not, what is preventing him or her from using them?

This provides information on pervasive and persistent beliefs about the self and others that might be core beliefs, as well as indicating the type of coping strategies that the patient usually employs.

When this information has been gathered, the patient and the therapist can work together to develop a conceptualization, perhaps using the conceptualization worksheet (see Figure 12.1). The developmental conceptualization includes the following:

1. significant life experiences, particularly early experiences
2. core beliefs about the self, the world (including illness and death), and others
3. rules and conditional beliefs (both general and illness related)
4. coping/compensatory strategies arising from these beliefs
5. cancer, or experiences related to it, as the critical incident
6. how the patient's beliefs and strategies are challenged by cancer
7. how the patient's current problems can be understood to arise from the way in which cancer challenges their beliefs and coping strategies.

Figure 12.2 shows an example of a completed conceptualization.

This conceptualization will place more emphasis on the role of the critical incident than in traditional CBT formulations. As we have seen throughout this book, the critical incident might be the diagnosis of cancer, or its symptoms, or the meaning of treatment side-effects. Whatever the external event that has contributed to the patient's decompensation, it is important to understand how it fits into their overall belief system.

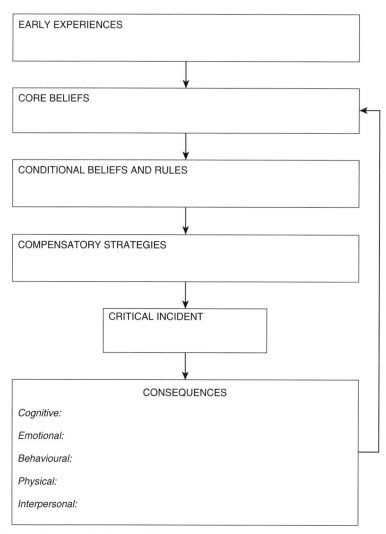

Fig. 12.1 Conceptualization worksheet.
Feeling Good: The New Mood Therapy by David D. Burns, M.D. Copyright © 1980 by David D. Burns, M.D. Reprinted by permission of HarperCollins Publishers.

Four ways in which life-threatening illness interacts with beliefs

1. Positive beliefs and coping are challenged

Many people are effective copers and have weathered many storms in their lives, but coping with a disease that might kill them is a different matter, and

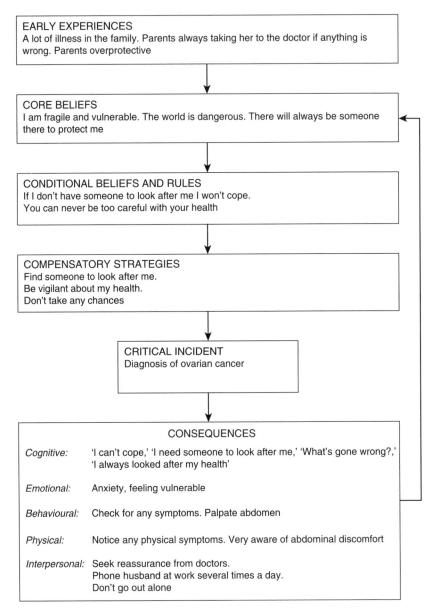

Fig. 12.2 A completed conceptualization for a 63-year-old woman with ovarian cancer.

Feeling Good: The New Mood Therapy by David D. Burns, M.D. Copyright © 1980 by David D. Burns, M.D. Reprinted by permission of HarperCollins Publishers.

for some time at least there will be doubts in everyone's mind. Will I be able to cope? How will others see me? Will I get the help that I need? Will I recover? Most people have remarkable resilience and bounce back. Our experience has been that identifying the patient's strengths and resources and remembering how they coped with past challenges often helps to turn a vicious circle into a virtuous circle. Work with these patients is about helping them to process what has happened and then access their old style of thinking and coping.

2. Rigid beliefs are shattered

Core beliefs that the world is safe, that one is safe, or that everything will turn out well can be undermined by a serious illness. The shock of the discovery that the world is not as benign as one had thought takes time to process, so again part of the work here is to facilitate a grieving process. There may also be conditional beliefs that can be identified and worked with (e.g. 'If I'm a good person, bad things won't happen to me'). This may be an opportunity for the person to learn from the experience and to experiment with more balanced beliefs (e.g. 'The world is generally a safe place, but bad things happen, and when they do I have the capacity to cope and to find help and support').

3. Ability to cope is challenged and underlying negative beliefs are confirmed

Here we find that negative core beliefs have been mitigated by conditional beliefs and compensatory strategies, but some aspect of cancer has acted as a critical incident and challenged the assumptions. An example of this might be a boy who grows up in a family where academic success is valued, but he is not a good scholar. He forms a core belief that he is not good enough, but discovers that he is very good at sports and wishes to have a career as a professional footballer. He is still not sure that his family rate him for this, but the compensatory belief 'If I can excel at sport I will be worthwhile' helps to keep his doubts at bay. When he is diagnosed with a sarcoma of the leg and has to undergo a below-knee amputation, his compensatory strategy can no longer apply. His beliefs that he is worthless are confirmed, and he becomes depressed. The developmental conceptualization can be used, as described above, to understand the impact of cancer, and patients can be helped to learn to evaluate the helpfulness of compensatory beliefs and behaviours, both by guided discovery and by experimenting with new beliefs and behaviours.

4. Pervasive negative beliefs are confirmed

Patients with chronic low self-esteem or those with personality disorder have core beliefs that are active for most of the time. These schemas operate like filters which select aspects of the environment that confirm the negative view and exclude information that disconfirms it. This applies to cancer in the same way as it does to all other areas of life, so the patient will automatically start to weave stories that incorporate cancer into their negative world view. For instance, a woman with a dependent personality may believe that she is incompetent and cannot survive without help. A recurrence of breast cancer is then seen as further evidence of how difficult life really is, and that she cannot realistically be expected to cope alone without considerable support from relatives and staff. Changing these core beliefs in short-term therapy is not realistic. The conceptualization can help the patient to make sense of their experience. They can learn to recognize the schema when something activates it (e.g. receiving an electricity bill may generate thoughts such as 'This is all too much. I don't know what to do. Why doesn't somebody do this for me?'), and learn to decentre from the thoughts and feelings. Relaxation and other mood regulation techniques may help them to weather the immediate storm when their core beliefs create strong emotional reactions. The conceptualization can be used to

Table 12.1 Effect of cancer on underlying beliefs and coping strategies

Beliefs and coping strategies	Effect of cancer	Management
Mix of positive and negative beliefs with generally adaptive coping	Positive beliefs are challenged, but strengths and resources are available	Facilitate emotional processing Identify and encourage previously effective coping strategies
Overly rigid positive beliefs	Assumptions are shattered	Facilitate emotional processing Identify and evaluate rigid assumptions Facilitate development of more balanced beliefs
Latent negative core beliefs with compensatory beliefs and strategies	Compensatory beliefs and strategies are challenged, and core beliefs come to the fore	Use developmental conceptualization to understand the impact of cancer Evaluate the helpfulness of compensatory beliefs and behaviours Experiment with new beliefs and behaviours Facilitate new compensatory behaviours
Negative core beliefs present most of the time	Confirmation of negative beliefs	Use developmental conceptualization to understand the impact of cancer Use decentring and emotion regulation techniques to help the patient to tolerate 'schema activation' Focus on coping in the here and now

identify what behaviours in the here and now are arising from the schema and maintaining the problem. Thus although the belief 'I'm helpless and incompetent' is not addressed directly, the strategy of clinging and constantly seeking reassurance can be worked with. For example, an agreement could be made between the patient and her partner that she will experiment with seeking less reassurance, and he will refrain from giving it. Table 12.1 summarizes the four ways in which cancer interacts with beliefs.

Working with assumptions and core beliefs

Testing assumptions can form part of the end phase of APT, together with preparations for ending therapy and relapse prevention work.

When these 'deeper' assumptions have been identified, cognitive and behavioural techniques can be used to evaluate them in the same way as we work with 'surface' cognitions. Approaches such as looking at evidence contrary to the belief, weighing up the advantages and disadvantages, etc., can all play a part in this process. Behavioural experiments can be especially useful for testing conditional beliefs. For instance, a patient who believes that she must look after people in order to make her life worthwhile was helped to identify the positive and negative consequences of this rule:

Positive consequences	Negative consequences
I'm always needed	I don't get time for myself
I can always keep myself busy	Sometimes I do things because I think people need them doing, not because they really need them
I can feel proud of what I do	My family don't get a chance to take responsibility for themselves
	I get cross if people aren't grateful
	When I can't do things for people (because of my illness) I get depressed

Having established the disadvantages of the assumption, the next step is to create an alternative, more healthy belief (e.g. 'If I respect others and myself, they will grow and I will grow'). This patient then devised new ways of behaving, to test whether this new rule applies. Experiments included refraining from always jumping in to bail out her son when he had spent all of his money, as well as asking people what they would like rather than acting on her assumption that she knows what they want, and scheduling time for herself. Framing the belief in the conditional 'If … then …' format allows experiments to be set up to test it. Framing a new adaptive belief in this way also allows experiments to be done that are actively testing something positive, rather than merely disconfirming a negative belief. These beliefs are often deeply ingrained, and they cannot be changed dramatically in short-term therapy. If they are addressed at the end of therapy, the patient will hopefully have gained insight into the 'If … then …' rules that he or she uses, and will also have learned strategies for continuing the work of challenging these maladaptive rules beyond therapy. As we have seen, core beliefs are not usually challenged directly, but these unconditional ideas about the self, the world, and other people can often be discussed openly with patients, and strategies devised for future self-help work.

Working with beliefs about illness

Maladaptive beliefs about illness and adversity contribute to the patient's distress and can interfere with medical treatment. The woman who believed that every time she got up she would be knocked down again ('If I get too cocky I will be punished for it') benefited from cognitive and behavioural interventions. Guided discovery revealed that there had in fact been some occasions on which she had been hopeful and things had gone well. She was also able to recognize that her belief was quite superstitious. The therapist then suggested a behavioural experiment in which this patient spent a day thinking the worst and then a day predicting the best that could happen. She recorded how she felt and what actually occurred. As a result of the experiment, the patient was able to see that good and bad things happened regardless of her attitude, and that although she felt quite tense and apprehensive when thinking positively, this anxiety decreased over the two days of the experiment. Although direct work on underlying assumptions is best left to the later stages of therapy, when the patient is less distressed and a full conceptualization has been developed, it may sometimes be appropriate to start to address beliefs about illness quite early on in therapy, because these beliefs may interfere with medical treatment.

Summary

As a short-term therapy, APT is not designed to promote personality change, but understanding how experiences shape core beliefs and the conditional assumptions and compensatory behaviours that arise from them may be helpful both to the therapist when planning treatment, and to the patient. A developmental conceptualization helps the patient to understand their reaction to cancer in a broader context, and can have a containing effect. Recognizing how the disease or its treatment has interacted with their beliefs to create the idiosyncratic meaning of cancer for this particular individual provides a valuable way in to understanding why the patient is distressed, as well as a way out of that distress.

Chapter 13

Working with couples

The problems of living with cancer affect not only the patient but also their immediate family, particularly their partner. The needs of family members have been increasingly recognized in recent years, and this is a growing area of research. Early systematic studies confirmed the clinical impression of undisclosed psychological morbidity in partners of cancer patients (e.g. Lichtman and Taylor, 1986; Moynihan, 1987). Similar factors appear to predict morbidity both in patients and in their partners, namely lack of social support, uncertainty, and hopelessness and distress about symptoms (Northouse et al, 1996). Psychological disturbance in the partner has a detrimental effect on the patient. Not surprisingly, the quality of the relationship also influences the patient's well-being. Partners who have a more affiliative relationship (Fuller and Swenson, 1993) or who are actively helpful (Pistrang and Barker, 1995) aid the promotion of well-being. Mellon et al (2006) interviewed cancer patients and family members 1 to 6 years after the diagnosis. Patients reported better quality of life, less fear of cancer recurrence, and more support than their family caregivers. Social support predicted quality of life in both groups. However, for the cancer survivors, family stressors, meaning of the illness, and employment status predicted quality of life, whereas fear of recurrence was the strongest predictor of family caregivers' quality of life. A range of couple-based therapies are available. Zaider and Kissane (2010) have reviewed their effectiveness for early-stage breast and prostate cancer and later-stage cancer.

The main purpose of including the patient's partner in APT is to ameliorate psychological distress in both partners in the relationship. This can be achieved primarily by enhancing the quality of the relationship. If the relationship is already strong, the partner can act as a 'co-therapist', helping in particular with cognitive and behavioural assignments outside the session.

Not all patients wish their partner to be included in therapy; some prefer to explore their feelings and cancer-related problems alone with the therapist. Clearly, the patient's wishes are paramount. During the first APT session, the possibility of including the partner is raised with the patient and, if the patient agrees, the partner is invited to take part in subsequent sessions. We adopt a flexible approach, enabling the patient and their partner to decide how many joint sessions they wish to have.

In this chapter we shall discuss the following:

◆ how to facilitate open communication between the patient and their partner

◆ the nature of relationship schemas in cancer

◆ basic cognitive techniques for working with couples

◆ examples of couples problems and how to deal with them

◆ ways to engage the partner as a co-therapist

◆ methods for treating sexual dysfunction.

Encouraging open communication

It should be noted that in the majority of cases, intimate relationships are not impaired by the experience of cancer. Indeed, some relationships actually improve as the trauma of cancer brings the patient and their partner closer together (Morris et al, 1977; Hughes, 1987; Zucchero, 1998). However, as was discussed in Chapter 1, there is evidence of deterioration of intimate relationships in a substantial minority of patients. A major cause of such deterioration is lack of communication between the patient and their partner (Lichtman and Taylor, 1986). In a study of couples where the woman was newly diagnosed with breast cancer, Hilton (1994) identified three major patterns of discussion about fears and doubts. In the first the couple were in agreement that talking openly was the best policy, in the second couples agreed not to discuss the illness with each other, while in the third the two partners held differing views about openly talking about their feelings. It was this last group which showed more problems in communication. Selective open disclosure was perceived as the most satisfactory pattern. Some barriers to communication have been described by Wortman and Dunkel-Schetter (1979). Patients and their partners often adopt a cheerful facade that belies the way they really feel. The responses of partners are determined by feelings of fear about cancer and the belief that they must appear cheerful and optimistic. As a result, the partner may show discrepancies between word and deed, encouraging the patient verbally while at the same time avoiding any discussion about cancer, or even avoiding the patient. The effect on the patient is likely to be a sense of rejection and loss of self-esteem. In order to regain the partner's sympathy and love, the patient may then attempt to suppress all of their negative feelings associated with cancer.

Encouraging the expression of thoughts and feelings about cancer

In order to overcome these barriers to communication, it is essential to encourage both partners to express freely all of their feelings, including anger, fear, and sadness. The techniques described in Chapter 7 can be used to facilitate emotional expression. We usually begin by asking the patient with cancer to talk about how they feel. Having learned how the patient really feels, the partner is then encouraged to express their feelings openly in the same way. The patient is often surprised to find that behind the partner's cheerful facade there is anxious concern and sadness. This discovery can be proof to the patient of how much their partner cares. Moreover, it may make the patient feel less helpless and more in control, as they can now do something to help and comfort the partner.

Listening and empathic communication

When emotional communication is initiated by the therapist in this way, it usually allows the couple to share their doubts and fears constructively. If they communicated effectively in the past, the obstacles set up by the cancer may be broken down, and they can go on to talk about their feelings together outside the session. However, some couples may not have been very good at talking even before the illness was diagnosed. In this case, both partners need to practise listening as well as expressing their feelings within the therapy session. Signs that more work needs to be done on communication skills training include the following:

- one partner interrupts or talks over the other (e.g. because they have difficulty tolerating strong emotions, or because they need to control their partner)
- one partner tells the other what they are feeling (mind reading)
- expression of feelings involves recrimination or blame of the other partner
- both partners talk at the same time.

The therapist asks the couple to take it in turns to describe their thoughts and feelings to each other. The partner who is listening is instructed to ask questions so that they get as clear an understanding as possible of what their partner is experiencing (by tuning into their wavelength). They are shown how to reflect back empathically by means of non-verbal gestures, by repeating and paraphrasing the partner's words (thought empathy), and by feeding back what they understand of their partner's feelings (feeling empathy). The therapist may need to initially model how to listen and reflect, and then allow the couple to try this out. The partner who has been expressing their feelings can then give feedback on whether or not they felt heard and understood. After the feedback the exercise can be repeated.

Communication training of this kind can be particularly helpful for the partner of the cancer patient who may be tempted to control, undermine, or invalidate the patient's experience, often with the best possible intentions. Simonton et al (1978) stated that 'the single most important thing the family can offer is the willingness to go through this experience with the patient.' One danger is responding by making the patient too dependent:

Patient:	'I'm afraid of the treatment. I really don't want it. I don't think it will help me.'
Babying reply:	'Now you know you've got to take it. It won't hurt you. It's good for you. And that's all we're going to hear about it.'

Simonton et al (1978) suggested an alternative reply:

Supportive reply:	'I know how you feel. The treatment scares me, too, and I don't really understand all that's involved. But we're in this together, and I'll go through it with you and help as much as I can.'

The patient and their partner may need to allocate time to talk and practise listening in this way as a homework assignment.

Cognitive techniques

Relationship schemas

As we have discussed in previous chapters, we all bring to relationships certain assumptions and expectations which are derived from our past experience. We have tacit rules about the way families should behave which we learn from our own families as children. These usually reflect cultural and social norms, but each family has its own idiosyncratic rule system as well. Cultural stereotypes include beliefs such as 'A woman's place is in the home.' Idiosyncratic family rules are much more variable, and include beliefs such as 'Parents should do everything they possibly can for their children at all times' or 'Parents should expect their children to do things for themselves or they will never stand on their own two feet.' These rules are rarely discussed. They are expectations of how things ought to be. One of the most important sets of beliefs are those about illness and how the family should respond to it (Williams, 1997). If the patient and the partner have different beliefs, this can lead to difficulties. These beliefs often involve assumptions about how the cancer patient and family members should think, feel, and behave:

Differing assumptions about attitudes to cancer	
You should *always* think positively	You should expect to feel sad all the time if you have cancer

Differing assumptions about emotional expression	
It's better not to talk about your feelings	You should let your feelings out as much as possible
Expressing feelings is a sign of weakness	Expressing negative emotions is natural

Differing assumptions about illness-related behaviour	
When you are ill you should let the family take over for you	I have to be a perfect mother even if I am ill
If I go back to work too quickly, that might bring the cancer back	Everything has to return to normal as soon as possible

If family members do not verbalize these beliefs, they will assume that others in the family are using the same rules. They then misinterpret each other's behaviour, making inaccurate attributions about people's motives. For instance, if the partner of a woman with cancer believes that it is a sign of weakness to express strong feelings, he may not indicate how upset he is by what has happened. She in turn may interpret his stoicism as a sign that he doesn't care. Cases 1 and 2 below demonstrate how misinterpretations and invalid assumptions can lead to relationship difficulties.

When the quality of a relationship has been poor for some time, maladaptive beliefs and behaviours become solidified. Attributions about the causes of the partner's behaviour become global and generalized. Failure to remember something is ascribed to stupidity, an irritable outburst is put down to bloody-mindedness, and feeling too tired to do the housework is viewed as a sign of laziness. These rigid schemas form a template which leads the couple to constantly look out for information that confirms their negative views of each other, and to ignore information that does not fit with the schema. Cases 3 and 4 below show how negative schemas can create a very skewed picture of partners' behaviour.

Challenging misinterpretations

The first step is to undertake a cognitive behavioural analysis of the couple's problem interaction(s). The therapist asks each partner separately for their view of the interaction, what they thought, what they did, what their partner did, and what this meant to them. The interaction can be drawn on a piece of paper or on a whiteboard (see Figure 13.1).

Case 1

After having a mastectomy a young woman lost interest in sex. She felt depressed and lethargic, and her negative thoughts centred on her disturbed body image: 'I am so completely unattractive that he can't possibly want me any more.'

When her husband made a sexual approach she rebuffed him, thinking 'He's only being sympathetic, he can't really want me.' Unaware of her automatic thoughts, her husband became prey to thoughts of his own: 'Her sexual feelings have disappeared. She's frigid.' He gave up making sexual advances.

Simply drawing this diagram may be sufficient to allow the couple to correct their misperceptions. If further work is needed, the next step might be to identify the cognitive distortions involved. Case 1 demonstrates a common cognitive

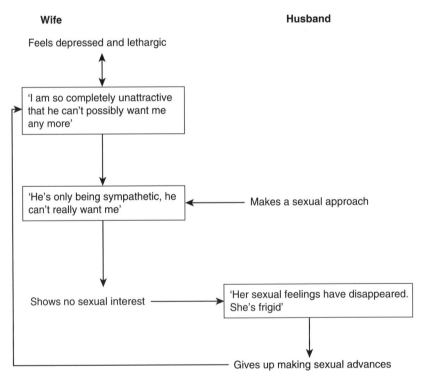

Fig. 13.1 Cognitive behavioural analysis of the interaction between the patient and her husband in Case 1.

distortion known as *arbitrary inference*. Each of the partners assumes that they understand the motives behind the other's actions, but they get it wrong. This 'mind-reading' bias can be discussed with the couple, and the disadvantages of jumping to conclusions can be identified.

In some cases it may be necessary to use cognitive techniques to evaluate the couple's thoughts and beliefs. All of the standard methods, including reality testing, searching for alternatives, etc. (see Chapter 9), can be applied. When interpersonal rules are identified, the costs and benefits of living by these rules can be explored.

Case 2

A woman with cancer had always been the dominant partner in the relationship. Her husband was a baker who worked very hard. He would come home after a day at work expecting his dinner to be ready. He found it difficult to cope with his wife's dependence, while she felt rejected by his anger. Both partners were using characteristic cognitive distortions.

Husband:	If you're not in hospital any more, you must be well (*all-or-nothing thinking*).
Patient:	He doesn't love me any more (*arbitrary inference*).

After helping the couple to reconstrue the situation, the therapist ends by developing an action plan with them. What can they now go on to do with this new knowledge? The couple in Case 1 might decide to spend some time together just cuddling and showing affection without engaging in sexual activity, to demonstrate to each other that each still cares about the other. Approaching intimacy in this non-threatening way could allow them to re-establish trust and so move on to re-establish their sexual relationship. The couple in Case 2 might agree on a compromise, whereby the wife does more as a way of showing her husband that she is active in her recovery, but he does more to look after her, acknowledging that he cares about her and that she is not yet completely well. When setting up behavioural assignments, therapists often use the principle of 'give in order to get.' When couples are resentful of each other it may be difficult to concede to the other partner, so setting up a contract where each agrees to do something for the other can feel more just. If there are two opposing positions, as in Case 2, the middle ground may allow both partners to feel that they are gaining something from the exchange.

In Cases 3 and 4 below we describe some ways of working with more entrenched relationship schemas.

Case 3

A young woman had unresponsive breast cancer. Her husband had sprained his ankle the day before. He asked her to take him to the shops to get some cigarettes, and she thought 'Why can't he go himself? He takes me for granted.' Rather than being honest, she retorted 'I'm not getting dressed yet, I may wait till this afternoon.' This caused her husband to escalate his demands and eventually force her to take him. It emerged that both partners had schemas concerning the other taking them for granted, and feeling unsupported. Therapy consisted of demonstrating the schemas, and encouraging more thought about what the other's perception of the situation might be. The other component of therapy with this couple involved finding more adaptive ways to express their feelings of being mistreated, without using emotive language that would inevitably upset the partner.

The final intervention with this couple can be undertaken on a behavioural level. The patient was constantly talking about cancer, and admitted that she had little time for anything else. The interactions in the relationship had become negative. Simply getting both partners to say what they like and then promoting an interchange of positive behaviours may help to improve the relationship.

Case 4

A woman with carcinoma of the cervix was being treated with APT for problems with anxiety. Early in therapy it became clear that she had a negative schema concerning her husband, whom she perceived as old, boring, and possessive (she was 50 years of age and he was 10 years older). This global negative view was so strong that she interpreted all of his attempts to support her in a very idiosyncratic way. He was keen to look after her and make sure that she did not overexert herself. However, she thought that this showed that he was treating her 'like a geriatric' because, being old, he wanted a 'geriatric wife.' When he asked her how she was feeling, she saw this as evidence that he actually wanted to keep her ill and dependent. This pervasive negative schema caused her to distort all of the evidence concerning her husband's behaviour.

Therapy attempted to focus on the marital problem, and in joint sessions evidence accumulated that the patient's husband was indeed concerned about his wife, and frightened. The patient refused to change her beliefs, which seemed to have been in existence long before the cancer was diagnosed, and APT was not successful. This raises questions about the effectiveness of APT when relationship problems are deeply entrenched. In retrospect, it might have been better to work with this woman on her own, focusing solely on her individual coping strategies.

The partner as co-therapist

Work on communication and cognitive restructuring is not required with all couples. If the relationship is good and the partner is supportive, he or she can be a helpful presence in the session, and can even act as a co-therapist. There are a number of ways in which the partner can make a valuable contribution:

1. by allowing the patient to express negative feelings in an atmosphere of acceptance
2. by participating in self-help assignments
3. by helping the patient to make decisions
4. by providing practical support when required
5. by encouraging and participating in joint activities
6. by helping the patient to regain self-esteem and control over their life by encouraging them to carry out those tasks and activities that are within their reach
7. by adopting a positive attitude towards the outcome
8. by providing information about past strengths, interests, and positive experiences which the patient may not be able to recall easily.

Treatment of sexual difficulties

There is documented evidence of impaired sexual functioning in a substantial proportion of patients with cancers of the breast (Wilmoth and Botchway, 1999), bowel (Devlin et al, 1971; Williams and Johnston, 1983), female genital tract (Wilmoth and Botchway, 1999; Jensen et al, 2004), prostate (Potosky et al, 2005), and testis (Rieker et al, 1985; Moynihan, 1987). The main causes of sexual dysfunction include the following:

- loss of self-esteem resulting from disfiguring surgery (e.g. colostomy, mastectomy), or feelings of being 'unclean' or contagious due to cancer
- physical effects of the disease (e.g. pain, bleeding, weight loss) and of cancer treatments (e.g. nerve damage in abdominoperineal resection), or fatigue, nausea, or hormonal changes induced by chemotherapy and radiotherapy
- cancer-related psychological disorders (e.g. depression, feelings of helplessness, anxious preoccupation with the disease and its recurrence)
- lack of communication between the patient and their partner (see above)
- pre-existing relationship or sexual difficulties.

The causes listed above are not of course not mutually exclusive.

Treatment of sexual dysfunction in the context of APT can be outlined as follows. A sexual history should be obtained from the patient and their partner as part of the medical/psychiatric history. It is important to enquire about sexual adjustment, as most patients will not reveal problems in this area unless they are specifically asked about them. Having established the presence of sexual dysfunction, the next question is whether such dysfunction is causing distress to the patient or their partner. In our experience and that of other researchers (Andersen, 1986), impairment of sexual function is not necessarily a source of distress to patients and partners. Clearly therapy is only indicated in those cases where sexual dysfunction is causing problems.

Therapy for sexual difficulties is based on cognitive and behavioural methods. Crucial to sex therapy is the encouragement of open communication and expression of feelings between the patient and their partner, as described earlier. Accurate information is provided to correct misapprehensions and to allay any fears (e.g. that intercourse can lead to recurrence of cancer). In this way, negative expectations about making love can be countered. Resumption of love-making as soon as is desired and medically feasible is encouraged. If intercourse is not possible for medical reasons, cognitive restructuring is useful, and ways in which the couple can re-establish physical closeness, and please each other sexually without engaging in intercourse, can be explored. Finally, for some sexual disorders, such as psychogenic impotence or vaginismus, the behavioural techniques of Masters and Johnson (1970) are appropriate.

Case 5

The following case illustrates how working with couples is integrated into the course of APT.

A 32-year-old man developed a painful swelling of his left testis. A stage 1 seminoma (early disease) was diagnosed and an orchidectomy was performed, followed by a course of radiotherapy. Despite being given an excellent prognosis the patient became increasingly depressed, and he was referred for psychiatric consultation 2 months after completing radiotherapy.

He had had a normal childhood, and he had one brother who had been successfully treated for a seminoma. There was no family or personal history of psychiatric illness. The patient had worked for 10 years as a car spray-painter. He had been married for 8 years, and had a 5-year-old son. The marriage was described as reasonably happy until a few months before the referral, when the patient's withdrawn and taciturn behaviour led to considerable estrangement. His wife described his premorbid personality as sensible, well balanced, and fairly passive.

The psychiatric examination revealed a 4-month history of increasing depression, listlessness, apathy, loss of libido, loss of interest, and insomnia. The patient felt unable to return to work. He showed some motor retardation, spoke in a low monotone, and was clearly depressed. He admitted to having some suicidal ideas. A diagnosis of depressive illness was made and fluvoxamine 100 mg at night was prescribed. However, the patient stopped taking this drug after only two doses because of its side-effects.

The patient was seen alone for the first session and together with his wife for five further sessions. During APT, the automatic thoughts of the patient and his wife were elicited. They were then taught to challenge these thoughts and to keep a daily record.

Patient

Automatic thought:	I'm not the same any more because of the cancer, so I won't be able to go back to work.
Rational response:	My fear of returning to work came from my *feelings* about myself since I got cancer, not from the disease itself. I have been told that I don't have any sign of cancer now and that my chances are very good.

Patient's wife

Automatic thought:	He's changed completely since he was in hospital. This cancer business has made him withdraw completely and, to be honest, I think he has stopped loving me.
Rational response:	Being told that he had cancer and having a testicle removed must have been an awful shock. It takes time to get over this.

The patient was urged to plan his daily activities and, in particular, to engage in those activities that would give him pleasure or a sense of achievement. Considerable collaborative effort was devoted to finding the patient's strengths and building on these. For example, after initial resistance, when he protested that he was unable to do anything at all, he was persuaded to take his son out to play football, and to decorate the bathroom. He found that these activities raised his self-esteem and were pleasurable. As a result, his mood began to lift. His wife reported that he was whistling in the bathroom, something he had not done for several months.

Communication between the patient and his wife was facilitated during joint sessions. His wife was able to tell him that she had become depressed as well as angry because he had withdrawn from her and appeared to have given up.

Before therapy, she had been unable to let him know her feelings because, in view of his cancer, she felt that she had no right to complain. However, she had expected him to know how she felt without having to tell him (Beck's arbitrary inference). The patient in fact had no idea how she was feeling.

Another issue which emerged was that the patient regarded his wife as excessively dominant, and thought that this was her nature and therefore unalterable. However, his wife did not wish to be dominant, but felt that she had been compelled to adopt this role by his unwillingness to make decisions ('He always leaves everything to me'). Through frank communication, the patient and his wife came to recognize and learn to overcome these problems.

The patient's lack of assertiveness had caused difficulties not only in his marriage but also at work for several years. He had felt angry because no precautions were taken against inhaling paint spray. He had never expressed his concern and anger, fearing that he might lose his temper and then lose his job as a result.

During APT, we rehearsed how he could express his concern appropriately to his foreman. He returned to work after a 5-month absence, just before completing APT. He managed to speak to the foreman and to politely insist on the need for facemasks to be provided. As a result, his self-esteem increased markedly.

Tables 13.1 and 13.2 show the effects of APT on scores on the Hospital Anxiety and Depression Scale (HADS), the Mental Adjustment to Cancer

Table 13.1 APT assessments of the patient in Case 5

	Pre-therapy	Post-therapy	4 months post-therapy
HADS	8	0	2
Depression	7	1	5
Anxiety	44	51	52
MACS	13	6	7
Fighting spirit	21	21	17
Helplessness	17	16	14
Anxious preoccupation	19	5	4
Fatalism	58	37	40
Rotterdam Symptom Checklist			
PAIS			
Total score			

HADS, Hospital Anxiety and Depression Scale (Zigmond and Snaith, 1983); MACS, Mental Adjustment to Cancer Scale (Watson et al, 1988); RSCL, Rotterdam Symptom Checklist (de Haes et al, 1987); PAIS, Psychosocial Adjustment to Illness Scale (Derogatis, 1983).

Table 13.2 APT assessments of the patient's wife in Case 5

	Pre-therapy	Post-therapy	4 months post-therapy
HADS	7	2	2
Depression	10	7	8
Anxiety	52	46	44
PAIS			
Total score			

HADS, Hospital Anxiety and Depression Scale (Zigmond and Snaith, 1983); PAIS, Psychosocial Adjustment to Illness Scale (Derogatis, 1983).

Scale (MACS), and the Psychosocial Adjustment to Illness Scale (PAIS) obtained by the patient and his wife. It is clear from Table 13.1 that the patient's anxiety and depression improved markedly, that he became less helpless, that most of his symptoms disappeared (as measured by the Rotterdam Symptom Checklist), and that his psychosocial adjustment (as measured by the PAIS, with lower scores indicating better adjustment) had improved. His wife's depression improved, but her anxiety remained much the same (see Table 13.2), and there was a slight improvement in her psychosocial adjustment. It is of interest that the improvement which was observed in both partners after six APT sessions was maintained during the following months.

Summary

With the patient's agreement, and where circumstances permit, their partner should be included in APT. Joint sessions should include some or all of the following tasks:

1. encouraging the open expression of feelings
2. facilitating communication between the partners
3. identifying maladaptive interactions
4. identifying cognitive distortions and challenging automatic thoughts
5. encouraging mutually rewarding behaviours
6. treating sexual dysfunction where appropriate.

Chapter 14

CBT in advanced and terminal illness

CBT is now increasingly used in patients with advanced cancer, and in palliative care (Mannix et al, 2006; Sage et al, 2008; Moorey et al, 2009). Throughout this book we have tried to demonstrate how cognitive behavioural techniques can help a broad spectrum of patients with different types of cancer and different life expectancies. In this chapter we shall consider some of the special issues that arise when treating patients with advanced disease.

In patients with early cancer, treatments may bring hope of lasting remission or cure, and following this there may be substantial disease-free periods. Psychological problems during this phase respond well to CBT. The negative thoughts that are experienced are often clearly distorted, and evidence is available to challenge them. The patient may have unrealistic beliefs about the effectiveness of treatment, the impact of side-effects on their life, or their ability to cope. Identifying and testing these beliefs by accessing appropriate information or setting up behavioural experiments is usually very helpful. Once the initial shock of diagnosis is over, it is not too difficult to help the patient to return to their old coping styles.

However, if the cancer does not respond to treatment, or if it recurs, the consequent demoralization presents a greater challenge. In advanced cancer there are three disease processes that can influence the patient's psychological response.

1. Disease may be present but dormant, or only growing slowly. Some people have the capacity to virtually ignore the existence of their tumour, without denying it. They selectively attend to the non-cancer aspects of their life. However, many patients find it frightening and frustrating to know that the cancer is still present. They cannot understand why it is not possible for it to be cut out, or why some treatment cannot be found to eradicate it. This leads to an anxious preoccupation with the current illness and its possible spread.

2. Progressive disease inevitably brings uncertainty about the effectiveness of further treatment, and about ultimate survival.

3. In some types of cancer, treatment is effective but does not bring permanent remission. This is common in myeloma and leukaemia, but may also occur with solid tumours. As recurrences mount up, it becomes increasingly difficult to maintain a fighting spirit.

It is not necessarily the stage of the disease as understood by the oncologist that is significant in determining the patient's emotional reactions, but rather the stage of the disease as it is understood by the patient him- or herself. Some people with advanced cancer may not have been told their prognosis, or may not want to know. Their reactions will be very different from those who are fully informed (e.g. those who know that metastatic breast cancer cannot be cured). However, it is not only the subjective aspects of cancer at this stage that cause variation in the psychological response. Different types of cancer, and even different forms of the same disease, can be associated with different prognoses. For instance, metastatic breast cancer involving the bones may be associated with much longer survival than metastatic disease in the liver or brain.

Advanced cancer refers to a broad range of patients. Life expectancy may range from 6 months to 6 years, and some patients may be experiencing severe debilitating symptoms while others will have no symptoms at all. It is therefore difficult to generalize about the relationship between advanced disease and coping. Classen et al (1996) studied psychological adjustment to advanced breast cancer in a sample of 101 women. As has been found in studies of early-stage cancer, fighting spirit and emotional expressiveness were associated with better psychological adjustment. Bloom and Spiegel (1984) found that avoidance coping strategies were associated with poor social functioning in women with advanced breast cancer. A few studies have made direct comparisons between the coping of patients with early and advanced disease. Greer and Watson (1987) found few differences between early- and advanced-stage patients in their responses to the Mental Adjustment to Cancer Scale (MACS). Both groups had similar scores for fighting spirit, helplessness, and fatalism. However, scores for anxious preoccupation were significantly higher in patients with advanced disease (see Table 14.1). Watson et al (1990) found that in a small mixed cancer sample, a belief in control over the course of the illness was associated with fighting spirit in early-stage patients but not in patients with advanced disease. A recent review of studies of positive attitude in advanced disease concluded that positive attitude and self-efficacy may be associated with better emotional adjustment, and that active, problem-focused coping appeared to be adaptive, whereas avoidant coping was maladaptive (O'Brien and Moorey, 2010).

Longitudinal studies of people with advanced cancer suggest that the majority of patients are able to cope well, but a minority become depressed with

Table 14.1 Mean scores on the Mental Adjustment to Cancer Scale (MACS) (Watson et al, 1988) for patients with early- and advanced-stage disease

	Early disease	**Advanced disease**	
Fighting spirit	52.3	53.1	NS
Anxious preoccupation	19.5	21.7	$P < 0.001$
Fatalism	20.8	20.0	NS
Helplessness	9.4	9.6	NS
Avoidance	1.9	1.9	NS

NS, non-significant. Probability was calculated using a two-tailed t-test.
From Greer and Watson (1987).

progression towards death. Lo et al (2010) assessed 365 patients with meta-static gastrointestinal or lung cancer at 2-month intervals. In total, 16% of these patients experienced moderate to severe depressive symptoms, which persisted in at least one-third of them. Moderate to severe depressive symptoms were nearly three times more common during the final 3 months of life than 1 year before death. Younger age, antidepressant use at baseline, lower self-esteem and spiritual well-being, and greater attachment anxiety, hopelessness, physical burden of illness, and proximity to death predicted depressive symptoms. Lo and colleagues observed that a combination of greater physical suffering and psychosocial vulnerability put individuals at highest risk for depression. Rabkin et al (2009) interviewed 58 patients with cancer on a monthly basis until their death. In total, 76% never reached the threshold for a depressive diagnosis, 3% were depressed throughout, and 14% became depressed for the first time during the study. Those who became depressed moved into the clinical range almost exclusively in the last visit before their death.

The psychological effects of physical symptoms

Despite these variations in the objective and subjective consequences of late-stage cancer, there are some factors that tend to distinguish it from early disease. One of these is the increased likelihood of physical symptoms from the cancer itself. In many of the cases that we have used to illustrate therapy, the patient was living an active life with few or no apparent signs of disease. In others, physical symptoms resulted from the treatment that they were receiving. Patients with advanced cancer may experience symptoms such as pain, breathlessness, nausea, and physical disablement. It would not be surprising if these caused more psychological distress in their own right, and the physical burden of disease does appear to be associated with an increased risk of depression

(Lo et al, 2010). However, 76% of patients with cancer never experience clinical depression during their last months of life (Rabkin et al 2009) In the cognitive model it is the patient's *interpretation* of the physical effects of the disease that causes distress. The symptoms of advanced cancer are often seen as a sign of permanent loss and a reminder to the patients that they will never return to their old self. This sense of loss may be associated with more global attributions about the self. Loss of the ability to carry out normal activities may be viewed as a sign of laziness or failure. These attributions usually imply a loss of self-worth resulting from the changes that cancer has brought. Patients with advanced cancer can feel like 'non-persons', as if they were being treated as if they were already dead. This is not surprising if the staff who are treating them, as Crary and Crary (1974) found, rate cancer as worse, less happy, and more worthless than death. Raising the self-esteem of the patient with advanced disease can be one of the most useful contributions of APT.

Burns (1980) describes the case of a woman in her mid forties who had disseminated lung cancer. She was weak from chemotherapy, and had to give up the daily activities that had meant a great deal to her sense of identity and pride. She wrote down the following negative cognitions:

1. I'm not contributing to society.

2. I'm not accomplishing in my own personal realm.

3. I'm not able to participate in active fun.

4. I am a drain and a drag on my husband.

Burns asked her to draw a graph of her personal 'worth' from the moment of birth to the moment of death (see Figure 14.1). She saw her worth as

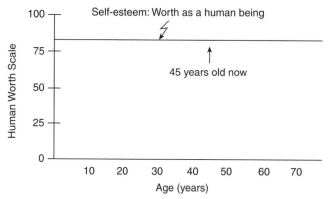

Fig. 14.1 Graph of human worth from the time of birth to the time of death, drawn by a woman with lung cancer (from a case described by Burns, 1980).

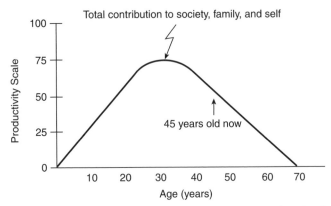

Fig. 14.2 Graph of productivity, in terms of total contribution to society, family, and self, from the time of birth to the time of death, drawn by a woman with lung cancer (from a case described by Burns, 1980).

constant throughout. He then asked her to estimate her productivity over the same period. This was presented as a curve with low productivity in childhood, increasing up to adulthood, and decreasing again later in life (see Figure 14.2). Two ideas then occurred to her.

First, although her illness had reduced her productivity, she still contributed to herself and her family in numerous small but nevertheless important and precious ways. Only all-or-nothing thinking could make her think that her contribution was zero. Secondly, and much more importantly, she realized that her personal worth was constant and steady. It was a *given* worth that was unrelated to her achievements. This meant that her human worth did not have to be earned, and she was every bit as precious in her weakened state. A smile spread across her face, and her depression melted in that moment. It was a real pleasure for me to witness and participate in this small miracle. It did not eliminate the tumour, but it did restore her missing self-esteem, and that made all the difference to the way that she felt.

This brief intervention proved very effective for this patient. Burns wrote that 'she died in pain but with dignity six months later.'

The concept of personal worth as a constant unchanging fact about the self may be useful for patients with advanced disease who have lost their self-esteem for similar reasons to the patient described by Burns. The next example shows how behavioural techniques can be used to combat the hopelessness that results from feeling incapacitated.

Cathy was a 75-year-old woman who had lived with cancer of the cervix for 12 years. She had had a tremendous fighting spirit, which had helped her through several major operations. She had great faith in the surgeon who had treated her over the years. Finally, the time came when further surgery was inappropriate and there was little likelihood that other treatments would be effective. In the past her doctors had told her what treatment she was going to have. Now they asked her if she wanted to have more chemotherapy. This left her feeling anxious and abandoned. She also felt very depressed and could not stop crying. The therapist helped her to express her feelings about the change of attitude of her doctors, and tried to help her to see that her tearfulness was appropriate and normal in the circumstances. She was very clear that she wanted to get rid of her depressed mood and return to her old self. When the therapist investigated the cognitions associated with her mood, it appeared that she was feeling ineffectual. She said that she could not lead a normal life, and therefore felt hopeless.

At the time of the interview Cathy was being fed intravenously and was quite weak. There was only a period of a few hours when she was well enough and free to walk about. Exploring what a normal life meant to her revealed a way in therapeutically. The therapist listed the activities that Cathy usually enjoyed, and then asked her which of these she could still do. The concept of all-or-nothing thinking was explained to her, and the idea was introduced that she could still do some, if not all, of the things that made up a normal life. She started a programme of gradually lengthening walks around the hospital, and scheduled reading and listening to the radio into her day. Her mood improved rapidly following this simple intervention.

A combination of cognitive and behavioural techniques is usually required to combat such hopelessness. Cognitive techniques help to challenge the thoughts that are paralyzing the patient. Monitoring automatic thoughts may show how cognitions such as 'What's the point?' precede the decision to stay in bed instead of getting up in the morning. Weighing up the advantages and disadvantages of doing nothing often leads the patient to admit that, whether there is a point or not, they feel better if they are active. Activity scheduling and setting tasks are the behavioural homework assignments that arise from this initial cognitive intervention.

Improving the quality of life

Improving the quality of life is the ultimate goal of all professionals who are working with patients with incurable cancer. Any palliative treatments must be measured against their toxic effects. Aggressive treatments that might be justified if there was a possibility of lengthening survival are not usually considered at this stage. Psychosocial interventions are part of the range of palliative treatments available to the oncology team. APT may be particularly applicable in this setting, because it puts so much emphasis on teaching the patient to plan and organize their time so that they can maximize their quality of life within the constraints of their disease.

Working with 'realistic' negative automatic thoughts

Many of the negative thoughts that are experienced by patients with advanced cancer have a realistic basis (e.g. concerning the possibility of treatment failing, or the possibility of death). Although these realistic negative automatic thoughts do not, at first sight, appear to be an appropriate focus for cognitive restructuring, there are several methods that can be used to help patients to deal with them (Moorey, 1996).

Understand the personal meaning

The first step is to understand the personal meaning of the thoughts for the patient. When dealing with death, pain, and disability, we all have memories and fantasies derived from our own experience of illness, which can easily get in the way of accurate understanding and empathy. Our own beliefs can create countertransference reactions (Moorey, 2010), where our schemas become enmeshed with those of the patient. Some common traps include being drawn into the patient's low mood or helplessness and hopelessness, and so concluding that nothing can be done, or working on the assumption that 'If I were in this situation I would feel depressed because I would be thinking ... '. Moorey (2011) has discussed how some of these therapist traps can be addressed. It is important that the therapist does not make assumptions about what the patient is thinking but that, as with all aspects of cognitive therapy, they check with the patient. This can sometimes be difficult because of their own anxieties about upsetting a patient by talking about death. However, since this is what has been on their minds, most people are not offended if they are questioned about the personal meaning of death for them. This can be introduced with a statement such as the following:

'Dying has different meanings for all of us. For some people it is the process of dying, for others the thoughts of who you will leave behind. Rather than assuming I know what you're going through, I'm interested in understanding what this means for you.'

Identify and test distorted cognitions using reality testing

Once the thoughts have been elicited, they can then be examined through reality testing. Evaluation of the evidence for or against these thoughts should be undertaken sensitively. Applying a rationality-based type of CBT in these circumstances can cause problems, because patients with incurable illness may feel insulted and invalidated if CBT is applied insensitively (Moorey, 2011). Therefore the thoughts that are tested in this way need to be selected more carefully in advanced disease than in early-stage disease. Misconceptions about illness, treatment, or pain control, and thoughts relating to guilt and self-blame or blaming others can often be dealt with using standard CBT methods.

Explore alternative perspectives

Many of the thoughts of patients with advanced disease are neither realistic nor unrealistic, and neither logical nor illogical. Because the patient is dealing with an uncertain situation, there are several ways in which that situation can be viewed. People who cope appear to see the glass as half full rather than half empty, and much of the cognitive work with patients with advanced disease involves helping them to explore alternative ways of thinking and acting. The key principle here is to find a way of viewing the situation that is helpful.

Examples of shifts in thinking that can be facilitated through discussion and questioning might include the following:

- deciding to be *life-centred* rather than *death-centred*
- deciding to focus on what the patient can control, not what they can't
- hoping for the best and preparing for the worst.

Linked to this is a decision about how much focus there should be on the illness and how much on other aspects of the patient's life (see below). A focus on illness and death can be valuable if it leads to either problem solving (e.g. making a will) or anticipatory grieving. However, if it is not focused on these it will just be rumination.

'Distraction', decentring, and defusion

The final approach to realistic automatic thoughts is to work with the process rather than the content of the cognitions. Reality testing and exploring alternatives both lock into the meaning of the situation, and it is easy to become stuck in a mode of trying to fix or resolve problems. Although some aspects of the life of people with advanced disease can be improved with problem-solving methods, many of them, particularly existential concerns, cannot. There is a danger that addressing these will encourage rumination (i.e. attempts to understand why this is happening, vainly going over the possibilities for cure, etc.).

Distraction or changing the focus to constructive activity

Throughout this book we have considered how changing the focus of attention can be helpful. This may take the form of distraction, but more useful is a decision to attend to life-enhancing or constructive activities that move the patient towards a valued goal. There is never enough time to do all the things that one wants to do in life. Knowing that one has a shortened lifespan highlights this even further. Doing nothing is not an adaptive solution to this problem. Organizing time, establishing priorities, and scheduling activities all contribute to the effective use of the time available and so improve quality of life. The patient's partner should always be involved in this process, as decisions about how the couple are going to spend time together are best made jointly. Involving the partner in activity scheduling can also prevent the inadvertent undermining of homework assignments by families who try to take over increasingly for the patient who is growing weaker and becoming less able.

Setting goals has another function. No one can tell a patient with advanced disease how long they have to live, only that their lifespan is considerably shortened. Deciding that they will be alive in 2 months' time and planning a goal to be achieved by that date is one way that patients can deal with this uncertainty. It can shift a future orientation that is focused solely on death into one that is focused on a life-enhancing event. Many patients spontaneously set themselves an important event in the future for which they will stay alive (e.g. a daughter's wedding, their own birthday).

Decentring and defusion

We tend to assume that our thoughts are reality. Cognitive therapy helps patients to gain perspective on their thoughts by examining them to see how realistic or helpful they are. This helps to create a distance, so that the thoughts are not at the centre of their experience and they are not fused with them. They learn that 'thoughts are not facts.' This is the central tenet of mindfulness-based cognitive therapy (Segal et al, 2002). Mindfulness practice gradually strengthens the person's ability to observe their thoughts and feelings without automatically becoming entangled in them. In Chapter 7 we introduced some simple mindfulness techniques that can be learned within APT. The techniques described in Chapter 10 will also be useful when dealing with worry and rumination related to advanced disease.

Promoting fighting spirit and positive avoidance

The different adjustment styles can still apply in advanced cancer, although they may not be manifested in the same form. Patients with advanced cancer still show a fighting spirit. Many people rise to the challenge of treatment failure and possible death by confronting it. The patient with a fighting spirit focuses on the quality of life available, and believes that they still have personal control. Sometimes this may extend to a determination to live as long as possible.

In advanced cancer the distinction between fighting spirit and denial may become blurred. A determination to beat cancer in the face of medical evidence that the disease is incurable could be said to demonstrate a strong fighting spirit or denial. Many patients show denial for at least some of the time during their final illness. The various ways in which the therapist can promote fighting spirit and positive avoidance in advanced disease can be summarized as follows.

1. The most optimistic prognosis available from the clinician is used to promote fighting spirit.

2. The therapist helps the patient to focus on what can be achieved in life, thereby maximizing their quality of life. This might be presented in the following ways:

   'You have tried the option of thinking about the future most of the time. What has been the result?'

   'What do you have to lose if you try spending more time on improving the quality of your life?'

   'We cannot increase the quantity of your life, but we can improve the quality.'

3. The techniques that are described in the rest of this book are used to promote activities which are unrelated to cancer, but important to the patient.

4. Cognitive techniques can be used to change the focus from what has been lost to what the patient still has (e.g. 'I may have cancer, but there are large parts of me that aren't affected by it. I will develop them to the utmost of my ability').

APT as part of palliative/hospice care

Fuelled by the emergence of the hospice movement in the late 1960s, the development of palliative medicine has led to major advances. Patients with end-stage cancer and other illnesses are no longer dismissed with a regretful shrug ('I'm sorry, but there's nothing else we can do for you'). Doctors and nurses now pay close attention to the physical needs and (increasingly) the emotional needs of patients who are nearing the end of their life, and continue to provide palliative care until death. Palliative medicine has received much less publicity and far fewer resources than the more glamourous medical specialties, but its impact upon the quality of life of patients with incurable illness has been considerable, and extremely beneficial.

The World Health Organization (1990) has defined palliative care as 'the active total care of patients whose disease is not responsive to curative treatment, where the control of pain, of other symptoms, and of psychological, social, and spiritual problems is paramount, and where the goal is the best quality of life for the patient and their family.' Finlay (2000) has provided a useful checklist of common problems in palliative care, which is summarized below:

Physical symptoms
Pain, nausea and vomiting, bowel problems, and other symptoms. A common and extremely distressing symptom is breathlessness (Ahmedzai and Shrivastav, 2000).

Emotional problems
Depression, anxiety, fears about the future, and responses to loss.

Social problems
Financial difficulties, stress in carers, loneliness, and work-related problems.

Spiritual issues
Unanswerable questions (e.g. 'Why me?', 'Is there an afterlife?').

Feelings of guilt about past events.

Family/carers
What do they need to know? What will the patient allow them to be told? Can they cope with the physical and emotional demands of caring?

For many patients with end-stage disease, palliative care is provided by hospices. It is a common misconception that admission to a hospice only occurs when the patient is about to die. In fact patients may be admitted on several occasions for symptom control or to provide respite for relatives who are looking after them at home. Hospices provide home care as well as treatment at the hospice, and palliative care teams that support patients and their families at home or in hospital are well established throughout the UK. Studies by Hinton (1994) and Morize et al (1999) have shown that during end-stage illness, anxiety and depression figure prominently among patients as well as among the relatives who are caring for them. In both groups these symptoms can be treated with APT. However, with regard to psychological therapy for the patient, close collaboration with physicians and nurses in palliative care is a prerequisite, as control of physical symptoms (e.g. pain, vomiting, dyspnoea) must be achieved before the patient can concentrate on and benefit from APT.

Terminal illness

Kausar and Akram (1998) studied 60 patients with terminal illness and 60 patients with non-terminal illness in India. Patients with terminal disease perceived that they had less control over their illness, used less problem-focused strategies, and used more emotion-focused and religion-focused coping strategies than patients with non-terminal disease.

The final stage of terminal illness begins when the patient enters a gradual decline and death is likely within a period of weeks or months. Many of the problems that are encountered overlap with those seen in patients with advanced disease, and similar psychological techniques can be used. A major problem for any CBT is presented by the increasing limitations that the disease causes. The more limited the scope for behavioural experiments, the more difficult it is to construct mastery experiments. Patients who have previously shown good adjustment to their disease and who have had a positive self-image can nevertheless become demoralized by the reduction in their functional ability. They may respond well to cognitive techniques aimed at showing them how their worth is not dependent on their ability to function. On the other hand, patients who have had previously low self-esteem or whose self-esteem is highly dependent on external factors such as their ability to succeed at work or to help others may not respond to cognitive techniques alone. Effective cognitive therapy involves cognitive change that is reinforced by behavioural change, which in turn produces further cognitive change. Clearly, the circumstances of terminal disease limit what can be achieved by APT. However, as described below, it is still possible to alleviate the emotional distress of patients and to do so without recourse to antidepressant drugs. It is important to remember that terminally ill patients under-report psychological distress, which needs to be elicited by means of skilled sensitive clinical interviews (Lloyd-Williams and Friedman, 1999).

Facing death

There is a dearth of systematic research on the experience of being close to death (Teno, 1999). This is hardly surprising in view of the daunting practical problems involved in undertaking such research. However, much can be learned from the comments of patients, as is illustrated below.

A dying man's thoughts
Have I given enough of myself?
Have I helped enough people?
Have I been kind in my life?
If the answer is yes,
Let me die in peace.

(Patient GM, 1970, personal communication)

I don't want my little boy to see me like this. ... I want him to remember me how I looked when I was well. I hope he'll remember that I loved him. I feel so weak, I haven't the strength to bounce him up and down on my lap. I just hope Charlie and my mum will look after him properly. If I know that, I can die in peace.

(Patient B, 1998, personal communication)

So, once we have recognized the limitations of the magic of doctors and medicine, where are we? We have to turn to our own magic, to our ability to 'control' our bodies ... for people who have cancer, it takes the form of a conscious development of the will to live. ... One of the ways that all of us avoid thinking about death is by concentrating on the details of our daily lives. The work that we do every day and the people we love – the fabric of our lives – convince us that we are alive and that we will stay alive. ... In considering some of the talismans we all use to deny death, I don't mean to suggest that these talismans should be abandoned. However, their limits must be acknowledged. ... As much as I rely on my talismans – my doctors, my will, my husband, my children, and my garden peas – I know that from time to time I will have to confront what Conrad has described as 'the horror.' I know that we can – all of us – confront that horror and not be destroyed by it, even to some extent be enhanced by it. ... It astonishes me that having faced the terror, we continue to live, even to live with a great deal of joy. ... We will never kill the dragon. But each morning we confront him. Then we give our children breakfast, perhaps put a bit more mulch on the peas, and hope that we can convince the dragon to stay away for a while longer.

(Trillin, 1981)

Main fears of dying patients

These include the following:

+ fear of the process of dying (e.g. intolerable pain)
+ fear of the consequences of death for loved ones
+ existential fear of death itself.

Identifying the cognitive processes involved in the appraisal of death is helpful. Many patients are able to express clearly what they are afraid of (e.g. 'I can't face a painful lingering death'). However, others find it more difficult. Careful questioning is then needed to establish which aspects of dying are most distressing. The most valuable information can often be obtained by asking the patient about the images they have of death (e.g. 'I can see myself deserted by all my friends'). Exploring these ideas and the feelings associated with them can be a painful process, but it sometimes allows the patient to clarify what they really fear and start anticipatory grieving.

Fear of the process of dying is by far the commonest fear, and is often due to distressing past experiences of watching a relative or friend with cancer die in great pain. Fortunately, there has been considerable progress in pain control and in the management of other symptoms in recent years (Turner, 1995), which allows us to reassure these patients. However, it must be acknowledged that certain symptoms of end-stage cancer, such as emaciation and weakness, do not respond well to the treatments currently available. Fear of the consequences of death for loved ones is an indicator of the patient's altruism. Such fears can be addressed in cognitive therapy in joint sessions with the patient and their loved one(s).

The existential fear of death itself is expressed in the question 'What will become of me after I die?' Any answer to this question will, of course, depend upon the individual's spiritual/religious beliefs. In his landmark study of dying patients, Hinton (1967) reported that those with a strong religious faith and those who were non-believers were least fearful about dying, whereas those with a faltering faith and doubts were most fearful. For patients who are plagued by religious doubts, referral to a minister of religion who is experienced in dealing with dying patients can be helpful. Of course, eliciting the meaning of death will depend upon the patient's willingness and ability to discuss the subject. Processes of cognitive and emotional avoidance can prevent thoughts and feelings about death from being acknowledged. Hinton (1967) describes how patients fluctuate between acceptance and denial, depending on how they are feeling and to whom they are speaking. Denial is not necessarily maladaptive in this respect. Hinton writes:

> Dying people are apt to speak or hint sombrely of the outlook at one time and talk lightly of hopeful plans soon after. Sometimes the hints that they give are fairly clear indications that they are aware of being near death. ... Sometimes spontaneous disclaimers of anxiety or deliberate avoidance of reference to the future, except in the vaguest terms, show that the outcome is suspected.

> (Hinton, 1967, p. 84)

The therapist must take the cue from the patient and work accordingly. Sometimes death may be an issue for discussion, while at other times the subject will be avoided assiduously. In these situations it may be best just to listen and offer support.

Few of us can face death with the apparent calm of Mozart, who wrote to his father:

> Since death (properly understood) is the true ultimate purpose of our life, I have for several years past made myself acquainted with this truest and best friend of mankind so that he has for me not only nothing terrifying any more but much that is tranquillizing and consoling!

> (Eissler, 1955, p. 000)

For most human beings, personal extinction is both frightening and unimaginable. When we are healthy, we live our lives without thought of death. However, when confronted with evidence of our mortality, we find it difficult to come to terms with the fact that, sooner or later, we shall cease to exist. A contemporary British philosopher has provided a vivid description of his feelings:

> I was overwhelmed, almost literally so, by a sense of mortality. The realization hit me like a demolition crane that I was inevitably going to die … as in a nightmare I felt trapped and unable to escape from something that I was also unable to face. Death, my death, the literal destruction of *me*, was totally inevitable, and had been from the very instant of my conception. … In the face of death I craved for my life to have some meaning.

(Magee, 1997, pp. 214–15)

It should be noted that Magee was not ill (terminally or otherwise), but was going through what he termed a mid-life crisis. The feelings that he so graphically describes are rarely expressed by people who are terminally ill. As was mentioned earlier, patients are far more likely to fear the process of dying and to be concerned about their loved ones. Indeed, death itself may or may not be a fearful prospect for the terminally ill. The individual's appraisal of death will depend on various factors, such as their personal circumstances, their spiritual/religious beliefs, and the degree to which adequate symptom control has been achieved. However, Magee's observation regarding the need to seek meaning in one's life is of particular relevance for patients with advanced and terminal illness and their efforts to cope. Folkman (1997) has demonstrated empirically that searching for and finding positive meaning is a crucial part of the coping process. There are various ways to create positive meaning (e.g. by making the best possible use of whatever time is left, or by finding that one's illness has strengthened the bond with loved ones or clarified which goals and priorities are important and which are not). For people with cancer who have young children, specific techniques for creating meaning include life-story books, letters to loved ones, audiotaped or videotaped messages, and memory boxes.

Another method of creating positive meaning is to set oneself certain goals. For patients with terminal illness, such goals may range from simple tasks which can represent an important achievement, such as being able to make a cup of tea or prepare a meal for their partner, to aiming to stay alive for long enough to see their daughter get married. The literature contains many examples in which a strong will to live or, conversely, the loss of will to live has apparently prolonged or reduced the duration of survival well beyond that expected on clinical grounds (e.g. Maguire, 1979; Selawry, 1979; Greer and Watson, 1987). Supporting evidence for these clinical observations comes from an epidemiological study that reported the postponement of death until symbolically meaningful occasions (Phillips and Smith, 1990). All of these ways of creating positive meaning are encouraged, and form an integral part of APT.

Case 1

The following case report illustrates the approach that is used in APT for patients with terminal illness.

> K, a 36-year-old French biochemist with testicular teratoma, was referred for psychological support. He had previously undergone an orchidectomy, chemotherapy, and surgical resection (debulking) of an abdominal mass in France. Despite this treatment, his disease was progressing, and the patient was fully aware of this fact. He had come to the UK to obtain further medical advice at the Royal Marsden Hospital.
>
> K was married with a 14-month-old son, and the marriage was described as 'stormy', with many arguments, particularly about money. At interview, K was understandably depressed and anxious about his future, and commented 'Do I have any future? I don't know.' He was also extremely angry with the doctors, who he said 'have put me through all this terrible treatment (chemotherapy) without any improvement in the cancer – do they really know what they are doing?' He was also angry with God for having allowed him to get cancer, as well as with his wife, because she did not show enough sympathy for him and she put their son first.
>
> Two main problems were identified during the initial APT session, namely the patient's inability to decide whether to have further chemotherapy, and the extremely disturbed marital relationship.
>
> In order to help the patient to make a decision about further chemotherapy, the therapist discussed with the oncologist the details of the proposed drug regime and the likely prognosis. The oncologist recommended an aggressive chemotherapy regime that would include cisplatin, and he estimated that the probability of cure with this regime was approximately 50%. This information was communicated to the patient, who was encouraged to consider carefully (in collaboration with the therapist) all of the advantages and disadvantages of resuming chemotherapy. K finally decided to accept this treatment, and was admitted to hospital.
>
> The second problem that had been identified, namely the disturbed marital relationship, was then addressed. A major obstacle was the absence of the patient's wife, who was living in France. She and K spoke on the telephone every day, and the content of these conversations was discussed during APT sessions. No major changes could be effected. However, some improvement seemed to occur after the patient agreed to put his finances in order and to make provision for his wife and infant son.
>
> When he was first seen, K asked the therapist to help him to develop a fighting spirit. This was done using the techniques described in earlier chapters. In addition, K was given a copy of *The Road Back to Health*, by Neil Fiore, to read (Fiore, 1984). This book seemed to be particularly appropriate for the patient, as the author describes his own recovery from metastatic testicular cancer. Unfortunately, it soon became evident that K was not responding to chemotherapy.

The goals of APT were then changed. The therapist discussed with K his feelings about active treatment coming to an end and the fact that death now seemed fairly close. The therapist asked him what goals he regarded as important for him to achieve before he died, and how he could be helped to accomplish this. K set himself the task of making financial provision for his wife and son. Fighting spirit came to mean retaining the will to live as long as was necessary to fulfil his aim. He achieved this, and was discharged from hospital to stay with his mother, who lived in London. A hospice team provided home care. K was offered continuing psychological support, but declined it. He died 2 weeks after being discharged from hospital.

Fighting and accepting

The above case illustrates the problem of adapting fighting spirit in patients with advanced and terminal illness. The active approach of APT in the early stages of cancer must be modified as the disease progresses. There comes a point when fighting to be cured or to extend life significantly becomes both unrealistic and counter-productive. Some patients are able to face this transition without too much difficulty. However, for many the thought of death is so terrifying that they try to keep fighting until the very end. Handling the transition from fighting to acceptance can be a difficult task. Kath Mannix, a palliative care physician who is also a CBT therapist, has suggested that one way to escape from the apparent dichotomies of fighting versus giving in and denying versus accepting is to reframe the whole process as *fighting for*. The aim is not to fight *against* death, but to fight *for* quality of life, and this can of course continue regardless of how much time is available.

When working with patients during this delicate phase, we suggest the following guidelines.

1. The therapist should work as closely as possible with the oncologist, so that both of them are clear about the prognosis and the available treatment.
2. The patient's wishes should be taken into account as much as possible. Acceptance should not be forced on a patient who is determined to fight, even if the odds are against them.
3. The patient's partner should be included in this final phase. The therapist must ensure that the patient and the partner are both agreed on the stance that they are taking against the disease.
4. The attitudes of the patient and their partner should be expected to fluctuate and not to conform to a steady pattern.

Renneker (1982) proposed that patients should be helped to fight to the end, to the extent of even asking physicians to prescribe placebo treatments. However, in APT the therapist takes the patient's lead with regard to the stance that he or she wants to adopt. Patients who continue to fight against death often experience increasing emotional distress. Around 74% of patients with an estimated survival period of less than 6 months report that they accept their situation, and around 9% report moderate to extreme difficulty with acceptance. However, the small number of patients who cannot accept their situation are more likely to experience clinical anxiety and depression (Thompson et al, 2009). For this reason, acceptance is preferable to fighting spirit during the terminal stage of cancer.

Case 2

Joan was a 60-year-old social worker who had advanced cancer of the lung. She and her husband would not accept the doctor's opinion that there was no treatment which could cure her. Her husband would say 'Why don't they give her hope?' Joan desperately wanted to hear good news, and would perk up if anyone said she was looking well. However, this only lasted for a short time, and she soon became despondent again. She was angry with God for punishing her in this way, and was very scared of death. None of the usual techniques of APT helped her very much. Focusing on quality of life did not work because she could not stop thinking about death. Allowing her to ventilate her feelings provided temporary relief, but in the long term only reinforced her resentment and despair. She refused to contemplate death, so nothing could be done to help her to face it. This woman's anxiety made the staff feel helpless. She continued to be distressed until she died.

However, such emotional distress, although common, is not inevitable in patients who fight to the end.

Case 3

S, a 65-year-old man with small-cell lung cancer, had undergone high-dose chemotherapy with autologous bone marrow transplantation. Despite this intensive treatment, which was accompanied by severe side-effects, there was no improvement in the cancer. He was told by his oncologist that no further curative treatment was available. However, S insisted that a new experimental treatment (which he had discovered on the Internet) should be tried. After discussions between the therapist, the patient, and the oncologist, the latter agreed to give the patient the experimental drugs. S put up with the unpleasant physical side-effects stoically. With the encouragement of the therapist, he planned various activities that were important to him and which he was still able to carry out (e.g. writing letters). His wife consistently supported him in his wish to 'fight the cancer.' S remained emotionally calm until he developed increasing dyspnoea. He died two days later.

Working with couples

We have previously emphasized the importance of including the patient's partner in APT. Although this therapy is aimed primarily at relieving emotional distress in the patient, including the partner in APT may also help the latter to cope after the patient's death. Where possible the therapist should encourage the couple to talk about death and the goals that they want to achieve before they are parted. Vachon et al (1977) reported that 81% of widows of cancer patients who had openly discussed death before their husbands died found that talking about death made it easier to face their bereavement. After the patient's death, it is appropriate to offer the partner bereavement counselling.

The following description of APT illustrates how therapy can be applied in a terminally ill patient.

Case 4

B, aged 28 years, was admitted to a hospice with breast cancer and liver metastases. She was referred because she had become severely depressed and refused to eat. When she was first seen she refused to talk to anyone. The therapist spent over an hour with her persuading her to speak. Eventually, with difficulty, she presented three main problems, namely feeling helpless, inability to eat ('I just can't eat'), and abdominal pain. Clearly, APT had to be integrated with palliative care, which required close collaboration between the physician, the therapist, and the nurses. First, adequate pain control was achieved within 2 days. Next, B's inability to eat was tackled jointly by the therapist and the nurses. As they explored this problem, it became clear that it had begun when eating was immediately followed by nausea. Although the patient's nausea had been successfully treated (with an anti-emetic), her inability to eat persisted. She was now able to challenge the automatic thought 'I can't eat' with the response 'The sickness has gone, so perhaps I can try to eat again', and the nurse was able to tempt her to begin eating small amounts of food. Finally, her feelings of helplessness were addressed. B knew that she did not have long to live. She felt angry that she would die so young, and she felt helpless about her 2-year-old son ('He won't want to see me like this … I can't do anything for him any longer'). The therapist challenged this negative automatic thought and suggested that B should test it out by asking her partner to bring her son to see her. Although she was reluctant at first, she agreed to do this. When her son saw her, he jumped on to the bed and put his arms around her. She became less depressed as she realized that, despite her illness, she could still be a mother to her son for brief periods.

Because she felt increasingly weak, therapy sessions had to be geared to her physical state and could only be brief (a maximum of 30 minutes). Nevertheless, B's psychological response was obvious. One major fear remained, namely what would happen to her son when she died. Her partner was not his biological father and had not legally adopted him. The therapist held a joint session with B and her partner. They agreed to legal adoption, and the next day a solicitor arranged this. B was encouraged to make an audiotape for her son. She died 5 days later.

Organic causes of psychological disturbance

Before we end this chapter, a note of caution is needed. Psychological disturbance can arise from the physiological effects of cancer itself or from the side-effects of opioids and certain chemotherapeutic drugs (see Chapter 1). Delirium (acute confusional state) is common in patients with advanced cancer, and especially in those with terminal cancer. This disorder, which is often mistaken for anxiety or depression (Levine et al, 1978; Breitbart and Cohen, 1998), requires urgent medical treatment (Greer, 1995). Therefore the therapist who is not medically qualified is advised to proceed with caution when commencing APT with patients who have advanced or terminal cancer. It is important to consider the possibility of an organic cause of the patient's psychological symptoms, and to request a specialist neuropsychiatric opinion if there is any doubt.

Summary

As an integral component of palliative care, CBT can be used to improve the quality of life of patients with advanced and terminal cancer. As the disease progresses, it becomes more difficult to conduct formal APT because of the patient's increasing infirmity. However, it is still possible to reduce their emotional distress by using the cognitive and behavioural methods that have been described in this chapter.

Chapter 15

Prolonged grief disorder among bereaved primary carers[*]

Psychological care for terminally ill patients does not end with the patient's death. Attention should then be focused on the needs of the surviving partner and, in some cases, other family members who were particularly close to the patient. A common fear among dying patients is worry about their partner (i.e. what will happen to him or her, and how he or she will cope). This fear, which can be extremely distressing for the dying patient, should be addressed by discussing it in a joint session with the patient and their partner, during which the therapist promises to be available for the surviving partner if required. I have found in clinical practice that such a promise is valued by the patient and their partner, particularly where joint sessions have been held previously. If, for practical reasons, the therapist cannot conduct bereavement counselling with every partner who requests this, referral to a trained bereavement counsellor can be helpful.

Most bereaved individuals cope with their grief without psychiatric or other professional help by means of various activities that tend to mitigate their distress. Such activities, which have been elegantly described by Colin Murray Parkes in his pioneering study (Parkes, 1986), include filling their lives by keeping busy, maintaining a belief that their deceased partners are (in a sense) still with them, and drawing on the support of family and close friends. However, a minority of bereaved people do not cope. They are stuck in a chronic state of mourning and seem unable to make the necessary adaptations to life in the absence of their partner (Prigerson et al, 2008), and they remain distressed by and preoccupied with the loss of their partner to the exclusion of everything else for many months, indeed often years. When these symptoms persist for more than 6 months, they form a clinical syndrome delineated by Prigerson et al (2008, 2009), namely *prolonged grief disorder* (formerly known as *complicated grief reaction*). The criteria for this disorder are listed in Box 15.1.

---

[*] This chapter is based on a paper published by Greer (2010).

Box 15.1 Criteria for prolonged grief disorder

A: Yearning (e.g. craving or pining for the deceased; physical or emotional suffering as a result of the desired but unfulfilled reunion with the deceased)

B: At least five of the following symptoms experienced daily or to a disabling degree:

1. Confusion about one's role in life, or a diminished sense of self

2. Difficulty accepting the loss and moving on with life

3. Avoidance of the reality of the loss

4. Numbness since the loss

5. Bitterness or anger

6. Inability to trust others

7. Avoidance of reminders of the reality of the loss

8. Feeling that life is empty and meaningless

9. Feeling dazed or shocked

C: Symptoms present for at least 6 months, and associated with functional impairment

Prevalence

The Yale Bereavement Study (Prigerson et al, 2008) consisted of a longitudinal study of bereaved individuals living in Connecticut, USA. At 6 to 12 months following bereavement a prevalence rate of prolonged grief disorder of 3.3% was reported. The authors have pointed out that this figure is almost certainly an underestimate, because the results were obtained in a particularly resilient population whose rates of mental illness were lower than those in other bereavement studies.

Further studies involving large numbers of subjects in different locations are required. However, regardless of the final figures, it is clear that bereavement results in serious and prolonged suffering for a substantial number of people. Bereaved individuals have poorer health outcomes than non-bereaved people (Stroebe et al, 2007; Lannen et al, 2008), and higher mortality rates are found in parents after the death of a child (Li et al, 2003), and among widowers (Parkes, 1986).

Risk factors for prolonged grief disorder

Ethical permission has been obtained to reproduce the clinical cases that follow.

It is widely recognized that the death of a child is likely to be the most traumatic event that a parent can experience (Sanders, 1979; Rosenblatt, 2000). The following is a poignant example.

Case 1

K, aged 46 years, was married but separated from her husband because of his morbid jealousy. She was the sole carer of her three children – a daughter aged 13 years and two sons aged 11 and 10 years. She stated that 'her world fell apart' when her daughter died suddenly as a result of a peanut-induced anaphylactic shock. K felt guilty about the fact that she was not with her daughter when she died, and she was bitter about her daughter's unsuccessful medical treatment and subsequent death. She could not accept that her daughter had died, and for months she continued to set a place for her at mealtimes, when she would talk to her daughter as though she was still alive. At other times she wept over her daughter's death and felt that she could not carry on without her. She pined intensely and continuously for her. Although she looked after the physical needs of her sons, she became emotionally detached from them. She felt that life had become meaningless. These symptoms had persisted for 18 months when she was first seen.

This clinical example has been included despite the fact that this woman's daughter did not have cancer, because she illustrates clearly the devastating effect of the death of a loved child. Most distressing for this mother was the fact that life had lost all meaning. Such loss of meaning has been vividly described previously (Currier et al, 2006; Neimeyer, 2006). The personal meaning of loss is a major area in CBT for the bereaved (Fleming and Robinson, 1991).

K's grief at the loss of her daughter was compounded by the fact that the death was sudden and unexpected. In these circumstances the bereaved person cannot prepare psychologically (i.e. anticipatory grieving) for the death of the loved person. Sudden unexpected death has been shown to predict poor bereavement outcome (Lundin, 1984). Conversely, a study has shown that individuals who were aware that their partners were suffering from a terminal illness more than 6 months before their death were significantly more likely to experience emotional acceptance during bereavement (Maciejewski et al, 2007).

Another risk factor, which is illustrated below, is a high degree of dependence on the person who has died (Johnson et al, 2006).

Case 2

F, aged 73 years, met her husband when she was 18 years old. He was 25, her first serious boyfriend, and they married a few months later. They had one son. F and her husband had a close relationship, but did not have any close friends: 'We kept to ourselves, didn't mix much, didn't need to because we had each other.' F was always shy, lacked confidence, and relied completely on her husband, who made all of the important decisions during their married life.

Two years ago, her husband developed a cerebral tumour (glioma) which led to increasing physical disability, blindness, and eventually dementia. F spent all of her working hours looking after him, with only occasional breaks when he was admitted to the hospice. Her son lived too far away to provide any practical help.

Following her husband's death, F, who was a practising Christian, became completely distraught. Life no longer had any meaning for her. She was angry and bitter, and commented that 'My husband's suffering was really cruel and terribly unfair. He was a kind, loving man who never hurt anyone. … Why should he have to suffer so much at the end?' She stopped attending church. Because she had been dependent on her husband all her married life, she found it extremely difficult to make any decisions. This in turn made the task of carrying out the necessary activities after his death onerous. She talked to her deceased husband every night, telling him how much she missed him and needed him. F yearned for her husband, and on several occasions she felt his physical presence in the house. 'Without Jack', she cried, 'my life has no meaning.'

Childhood Bereavement and Separation Anxiety

The converse of the death of a child, namely childhood bereavement due to death of a parent, is also likely to be a major risk factor. This particular topic has been described in detail by Beverley Raphael in her seminal work (Raphael, 1984), but is beyond the scope of this chapter, which deals with adult bereavement.

Based on a recent study of 283 bereaved adults, a statistically significant association was reported between complicated grief and separation anxiety in childhood (Vanderwerker et al, 2006). Childhood separation anxiety was not associated with depressive disorder, post-traumatic stress disorder, or generalized anxiety disorder. These results, if confirmed, indicate that a history of separation anxiety in childhood may be a major risk factor in adult life. Indeed, some leading authorities suggest that insecure attachment styles (Van Doom et al, 1998; Silverman et al, 2001; Grayling, 2002; Tomarken et al, 2007) in childhood are central to the aetiology of complicated grief (i.e. prolonged grief disorder) (Prigerson et al, 2008).

Case 3

B, a 61-year-old artist, lost her partner 16 months ago when he died of pancreatic cancer. The couple had been together for 29 years. Although their relationship was close, there was one serious recurring problem. B became distressed every time her partner went out alone to see his male friends or to go to his club. She did not suspect him of infidelity, but simply could not accept being left alone. She would cry and beg him not to leave her. This caused many arguments.

B was an only child. When she was 4 years old, her father left home. She became extremely anxious whenever she was separated from her mother even for a few minutes. She clung to her mother throughout her childhood and subsequently as an adult until she met her partner at the age of 32 years.

B nursed her partner during his illness, which began with indigestion, anorexia, and abdominal pain. He developed jaundice and eventually intestinal obstruction. Despite surgery and chemotherapy, his illness progressed, with weight loss and increasing pain, notwithstanding attempts at pain control. B insisted on bringing him home from the hospital, and she nursed him herself, with assistance from hospice nurses, until his death 9 months later.

When she was seen 16 months after her partner's death, B was bitter and angry, and felt that she could never trust doctors again. She yearned for her partner to such an extent that she was unable to resume her work as an artist or to see friends. Her history clearly reveals the role of childhood separation anxiety and insecure attachment style in her prolonged grief disorder.

Reported risk factors for prolonged grief disorder are listed in Box 15.2. It should be noted that evidence for these factors is often based on correlational studies. However, longitudinal studies are required to verify the reported findings.

Treatment of prolonged grief disorder

In the words of a contemporary British philosopher, 'The world is never the same again after bereavement. We do not get over losses, we merely learn to live with them' (Grayling, 2002). This opinion accords with our clinical observations. The aim of therapy is not to achieve so-called 'closure', but to enable bereaved people to learn to live with their loss. Thus the broad aim of therapy is to enable the bereaved person to find meaning in the midst of loss (Neimeyer, 2006).

The focus in this chapter is on prolonged grief disorder following a cancer-related death. This involves watching the slow, painful emaciation and eventual death of a loved person, which is clearly a prolonged and

Box 15.2 Reported risk factors for prolonged grief disorder

- Death of one's child
- Death of a parent
- Close relationship with the deceased
- High level of dependence on the deceased
- Insecure attachment styles
- Loss of meaning in one's life
- Sudden unexpected death
- Childhood separation anxiety
- Childhood abuse

distressing experience. Moreover, the grieving survivor often has doubts about the treatment that the deceased received, particularly the vexed question of any perceived or real delay in diagnosis. Such doubts will produce anger and increase grief, and must be addressed by the therapist.

Some useful guidelines

1. Before commencing CBT, the therapist should become thoroughly acquainted with the details of the deceased patient's illness and treatment.

2. The first step is to ask the bereaved person to give a detailed account of the months and weeks leading up to the death of the patient, and the impact of this on his or her life.

3. A personal and psychiatric history should be taken, including any evidence of childhood separation anxiety.

4. Cognitive and behavioural procedures are appropriate. The aims of therapy should be defined jointly with the bereaved person.

Cognitive techniques

It is important to look for and challenge any thinking errors. Common errors among the bereaved include the following:

- Unjustified guilt and self-criticism, often characterized by 'should' statements (e.g. 'I should have taken my wife to the doctor sooner, and if I had, she might be alive today', 'I should have been with him the moment he died, but I went to make a phone call and when I came back into the room he was dead').

It is important for the therapist to distinguish between self-criticism that is situation-specific (i.e. confined to events surrounding the loved one's terminal illness) and self-criticism that is symptomatic of a pervasive negative core belief. The latter is clearly more difficult to deal with, and requires more prolonged therapy during which the possible causes of such beliefs can be explored and challenged.

- All-or-nothing thinking (e.g. 'Since he died my life has ended').
- Negative predictions (e.g. 'I could never be happy again').
- Inappropriate anger directed at doctors and nurses who treated the dying patient.
- A fear that details of the partner's appearance or voice cannot be recalled precisely, and that the bereaved person will eventually forget the deceased. Reassurance is required from the therapist that even if certain details become hazy, the memory of the deceased will remain accessible.

Behavioural techniques
These include the following:

- Setting attainable, jointly agreed goals that give a sense of pleasure or achievement (e.g. going out with friends, gardening, settling financial affairs arising from the partner's death). Such goals encourage the gradual resumption of former activities. If, as often happens, the bereaved person feels guilty about deriving any pleasure from activities, reassurance can usually be given by asking whether the deceased partner would approve of such feelings.
- Daily activity schedules should be recorded and brought to the therapy sessions. The advantages of recording daily activities have been outlined in detail in Chapter 8.
- The emotional expression of grief should be encouraged.

Case 4

P is a 71-year-old retired engineer whose wife died of breast cancer 9 months ago. They had a happy marriage and decided not to have children. They enjoyed each other's company and shared several interests, as well as a sense of humour. Ten years ago P's wife developed a depressive illness during which her husband was supportive, helping her through this difficult period which lasted a year.

Her cancer, which was diagnosed 2 years previously, had progressed despite treatment with surgery, chemotherapy, and tamoxifen. She became increasingly fatigued and weak, lost 9 kilograms in weight, and developed painful bony vertebral metastases that eventually resulted in paraplegia. With the assistance of home care nurses from a hospice, and two brief admissions to the hospice, P looked after his wife at home until her deteriorating physical state meant that she required admission to a nursing home, where she died 10 days later.

During the 9 months following his wife's death, P developed classical symptoms of prolonged grief disorder. He yearned for her presence, felt intense grief, could not believe that she was dead, and felt numb and unable to get on with his life, which no longer had any meaning for him. He stopped seeing his friends and would not answer the phone. He described himself as 'empty, devoid of all feeling.'

Therapy began with attempts at *guided mourning* as described by Mawson et al (1981), whereby the patient was urged to recall and repeatedly describe in detail his wife's final illness and the circumstances surrounding her death. This procedure failed to produce any improvement. CBT proved more successful. The agreed aims of therapy were to relieve his intense grief, and to enable him to resume his previously normal life. P readily accepted the cognitive model as rational, which was important to him. Together with the therapist, he was able to identify and subsequently challenge a number of thinking errors (e.g. 'I failed (the deceased) because I should never have let her go to the nursing home – she didn't want to go', 'Perhaps if I had kept her at home, she would have lived longer ... maybe even still be alive'). These negative automatic thoughts plagued him, resulting in considerable guilt, self-criticism, and distress.

During the CBT sessions, P found that these distressing symptoms could be alleviated by challenging the underlying negative thoughts and adopting rational responses (e.g. 'It was impossible on medical grounds to continue nursing her at home, which is why admission to a nursing home was necessary', 'There was no evidence to suggest that she would have lived longer had she remained at home'). He had visited his wife every day for several hours, and agreed that the medical and nursing care was in fact 'first rate.'

The behavioural component of CBT consisted of setting goals that were realistic and attainable. He agreed that a reasonable task was to make and answer phone calls, but found that he could not do this. The reason which emerged during therapy was that he feared he would be overwhelmed emotionally if and when relatives or friends asked about his wife's death and his current feelings. The therapist suggested that P could control which topics he wished or did not wish to discuss, and this would remove his fear of being overwhelmed. He was encouraged to make a phone call to his sister, whom he least feared contacting. To his surprise, he was able to control the conversation as suggested. He then felt able to talk to other relatives and friends. As a result, he lost his fear, which was an important step in overcoming his social isolation.

However, P still spent much of his time sitting at home, grief-stricken, and doing nothing. He was asked to draw up a list of tasks that could provide a sense of achievement and/or pleasure, and to record what he managed to do every day in a diary (activity scheduling). He undertook a series of activities, ranging from simple tasks (e.g. planting bulbs in the garden) to difficult ones (e.g. sorting out his wife's clothing so that he could take it to a charity shop), which resulted in a gradual return to a more normal daily life. At the completion of CBT after 10 sessions, P was much improved. Although he continued to miss his wife and he mourned her, he no longer suffered from the symptoms of complicated grief reaction and had begun to resume his normal life. He had maintained his progress when he was seen at a follow-up 6 months later (see Table 15.1).

The use of CBT in prolonged grief disorder is a relatively new field. What is required now is the application of rigorous large-scale randomized controlled trials in which CBT is compared with other psychological therapies. A start has been made by Shear et al (2005), who compared 16 sessions of 'complicated grief therapy' based partly on cognitive and behavioural techniques with a similar number of sessions of standard interpersonal psychotherapy. The authors reported that their cognitive/behavioural-based therapy was significantly superior to interpersonal psychotherapy in reducing distressing grief symptoms. The other randomized controlled trial that has been published to date reported CBT to be superior to supportive counselling in reducing symptoms of prolonged grief disorder (Boelan et al, 2007). Treatment of people suffering from prolonged grief disorder is an important clinical task and one that should be evidence based, hence the need for further research into psychological therapies that are specifically designed for patients with prolonged grief disorder.

Table 15.1 Hospital Anxiety and Depression Scale (HADS) scores for the surviving partner P in Case 4

	First CBT session	End of CBT	6-month follow-up
Anxiety	11	6	5
Depression	15	8	7

Summary

The bereaved primary carers of cancer patients require psychological treatment if they are found to have developed prolonged grief disorder. The diagnostic criteria for this disorder and the incidence and possible major risk factors have been outlined. Some clinical illustrations have been presented, and treatment by means of CBT has been described, together with some clinical guidelines. The dearth of randomized controlled trials highlights the need for such trials of treatment.

Chapter 16

Group therapy

Individual versus group therapy

David Spiegel, a pioneer of group therapy for cancer patients, has proposed that group therapy has three advantages (Spiegel et al, 1999):

1. the social (i.e. emotional) support that patients give each other
2. the 'helper-therapy principle', whereby patients gain self-esteem through their ability to help others in the group
3. cost-effectiveness.

The last-mentioned advantage is of course self-evident. However, despite increasing pressure (both in the UK and in the USA) from those who hold the purse-strings and who know the cost of everything but the value of nothing, money should not be the deciding factor. We would agree that the first two advantages listed by Spiegel are undoubtedly important arguments in favour of group therapy. On the other hand, therapy that is undertaken with individual patients together with their partners (i.e. APT, as described by us) also has certain advantages. First, it is widely recognized that the effects of cancer involve not only the patient but also their loved ones (e.g. Baider et al, 1996), and it is important to involve the latter in the patient's cancer care (Speice et al, 2000). This is achieved with APT. Secondly, an inconvenient fact that is not mentioned in the literature on group therapy is that by no means all patients wish to join a group; some prefer individual psychotherapy. Indeed, there are often considerable difficulties in recruiting cancer patients to group therapy, and refusal rates as high as 69% (Ford et al, 1990) and even 80% (Edelman et al, 1999b) have been reported. Semple et al (2006) asked patients with head and neck cancer what their preferred form of CBT would be. They ranked individual therapy first, followed by bibliotherapy, and group therapy was the least popular option. The answer is clear – both individual and group therapy should be made available, and patients should be given a choice.

In Chapter 3, our review of clinical trials revealed that psychological therapy can significantly improve the quality of life (i.e. psychosocial adjustment) of patients with cancer, and such improvement has been documented in trials of both group and individual therapy. Direct comparisons of group and individual counselling are rare. Cain et al (1986) randomly assigned a consecutive series of women with gynaecological cancers to routine care, individual counselling, and group counselling, respectively. Counselling consisted of 8 sessions during which patients discussed their fears, were informed about their cancers, and were advised about diet, physical exercise, and sexual functioning. They were also given relaxation training, and were encouraged to express their feelings to caregivers and family, and to develop short- and long-term goals. Six months after counselling, patients in both of the counselling groups showed significantly improved psychosocial adjustment compared with controls. Individual counselling and group counselling were found to be equally beneficial.

Fawzy et al (1996) allocated 104 patients with newly diagnosed malignant melanoma to either 6 sessions of group CBT, 6 sessions of individual CBT, or assessment only. Again the group and individual treatments were equally effective, and both were superior to the control condition. At a 1-year follow-up the group treatment actually produced more improvement than individual therapy on a measure of coping skills.

In a meta-analysis of trials that sought to alleviate anxiety and/or depression in people with cancer, Sheard and Maguire (1999) found that group therapy and individual therapy were equally effective (see Chapter 3).

Different models of group therapy

Various kinds of group therapy that are run by professionals for cancer patients have been described. Psychoeducational *groups* focus on teaching patients about their cancers and the treatments that they are receiving. In addition, coping skills, stress management, and relaxation exercises are often taught. Therapy is brief, usually lasting for about 6 to 8 weeks. Examples of psychoeducational group therapy programmes that have been evaluated in randomized trials include studies by Weisman et al (1980), Johnson (1982), Cain et al (1986), Cunningham and Tocco (1989), Fawzy et al (1990a,b), and Berglund et al (1994).

Supportive-expressive group therapy has been developed by Spiegel and his colleagues (Spiegel et al, 1981, 1989), and details of the techniques used have been published in the form of a manual (Spiegel and Spira, 1991). In summary, groups of 7 to 10 women with metastatic breast cancer met weekly for a year. During these meetings the patients discussed their cancer treatments, family and communication problems, learning to live with terminal illness, and issues of dying and death. The emphasis was placed on expressing feelings and fears about their disease, and on mutual support and learning from each other – the so-called 'helper-therapy principle.'

Cognitive-behavioural methods have been adapted to meet the specific needs of patients with cancer in the form of individual therapy (Moorey and Greer, 1989), and subsequently in the form of group therapy (Kissane et al, 1997; Edelman et al, 1999b). The characteristics of individual therapy in the form of APT, which we described in detail earlier in this book, can also be applied in group therapy. These include focusing on specific current problems, identifying and challenging negative automatic thoughts, setting goals, developing coping skills, scheduling activities that provide a sense of achievement and/ or pleasure, relaxation training, and encouragement of the expression of emotions.

The three broad categories of group therapy described here are neither sharply defined nor mutually exclusive. In practice, clinicians sometimes combine elements from more than one type of therapy. For example, the group therapy described by Cunningham and Tocco (1989) combined psychoeducational methods with supportive discussions and some cognitive-behavioural methods. One apparent difference between the various types of group therapy is the duration of treatment. Psychoeducational and cognitive-behavioural therapies are usually brief interventions (around 6 to 12 sessions), whereas therapy in Spiegel's supportive-expressive groups was continued for a whole year. However, that study involved women with advanced disease (Spiegel et al, 1989). Spiegel et al (1999) adapted supportive-expressive group therapy for women with recently diagnosed breast cancer for 12 weekly sessions only.

Box 16.1 summarizes the techniques that have been used in seven of the outcome studies of group CBT for people with cancer. The most common interventions have been relaxation, monitoring and challenging of automatic thoughts, education about cancer, goal setting, problem solving, communication and assertion, stress management, and psychological support.

What group therapies have in common

Having described the different models of group therapy, it should be noted that they generally share certain important characteristics. These can be summarized as follows.

◆ The *mutual support* that patients give each other is the bedrock of all types of group therapy. One practical consequence of this is that, in contrast to group therapy in psychiatric practice, cancer patients are encouraged to maintain contact with each other outside the group sessions.

Box 16.1 Group CBT interventions that have been used for people with cancer

- Education about cancer (Heinrich and Schag, 1985; Fawzy et al, 1990a,b, 1993)
- Relaxation (Heinrich and Schag, 1985; Telch and Telch, 1986; Cunningham and Tocco, 1989; Fawzy et al, 1990a,b, 1993; Edelman et al, 1999a,b; Edmonds et al, 1999)
- Positive mental imagery (Cunningham and Tocco, 1989; Edmonds et al, 1999)
- Goal setting (Cunningham and Tocco, 1989; Edelman et al, 1999a,b; Edmonds et al, 1999)
- Physical activity (Heinrich and Schag, 1985)
- Scheduling pleasant events (Telch and Telch, 1986)
- Lifestyle management (Cunningham and Tocco, 1989; Edmonds et al, 1999)
- Problem solving (Telch and Telch, 1986; Fawzy et al, 1990a,b, 1993)
- Communication and assertion (Telch and Telch, 1986; Edelman et al, 1999a,b)
- Feelings management (Telch and Telch, 1986)
- Stress management (Telch and Telch, 1986)
- Coping skills training (Fawzy et al, 1990a,b, 1993)
- Monitoring and challenging negative automatic thoughts (Telch and Telch, 1986; Cunningham and Tocco, 1989; Edelman et al, 1999a,b; Edmonds et al, 1999)
- Psychological support (Telch and Telch, 1986; Fawzy et al, 1990a,b, 1993)

- The therapist focuses with the group on *current problems*.
- The therapist facilitates *interaction* between members of the group.
- The open expression of feelings is encouraged.
- Through the group process the therapist fosters the *development of active coping strategies*. This usually begins (as in individual therapy) with information and emotion-focused coping, followed by problem-focused resolution of patients' current concerns (Spiegel et al, 1999), and finally

the encouragement of meaning-based coping to promote psychological well-being (Folkman and Greer, 2000).

Therapy for all or selected patients?

Should all patients who develop cancer, or only those who show evidence of emotional distress, receive psychological therapy? A common-sense approach to this perennial question should be adopted. In our clinical experience (in the UK), cancer patients who show only minor or no evidence of psychological morbidity are, understandably, likely to decline invitations to take part in psychotherapy. The needs of these patients are best served by trained oncology counsellors, usually nurses, who will provide information or explanations as requested. By contrast, patients who need and are likely to benefit from psychological therapy are those who experience persistent emotional distress, who feel helpless and hopeless, and who are clinically anxious or depressed. Indeed the studies that have treated these high-risk groups appear to have achieved better results (Sheard and Maguire, 1999). Such patients can be identified by means of psychological screening instruments such as those developed by Weisman et al (1980), Greer and Watson (1987), Zabora et al (1990), and Watson et al (1994).

Practical considerations

When the decision has been made to set up a group therapy service, a number of practical issues need to be considered. How many patients should be included in the group? Should the group be open (i.e. new patients can join it at any time) or closed (i.e. once the group is formed and for the duration of therapy no new patients can join it)? Should patients with different cancers at various stages of disease be included, or should any given group be confined to patients with the same type of cancer and disease stage? At which stages during the course of cancer should therapy be offered? Finally, for how long should therapy be continued? No definitive, evidence-based answers can be given to these questions. However, there are several detailed informative descriptions of group therapy in the literature (e.g. Spiegel and Spira, 1991; Kissane et al, 1997; Spira, 1998; Edelman et al, 1999a,b; Feigin et al, 2000), which provide useful guidelines.

Therapy is usually conducted with 6 to 12 patients in closed or semi-closed groups. In both cases, patients commit themselves to an agreed number of sessions. Closed groups are more suitable for short-term therapy. However, where long-term therapy is planned (particularly for patients with advanced disease), the likelihood of a high drop-out rate due to increasing infirmity or death precludes a closed group. Under these circumstances, a semi-closed group to which new patients can be invited in place of those who leave is the best option. With regard to diagnosis and stage of disease, nearly all therapists (with the exception of Weisman et al, 1980) favour groups consisting of patients with the same cancer at a similar stage of disease. The advantages of homogeneous groups, whose members have much in common, are obvious. However, as far as uncommon cancers are concerned it may not be possible to find sufficient numbers of patients to form such groups (Spira, 1998). To overcome this practical problem, Spira advocates the use of mixed groups consisting of patients with a variety of cancers at various stages of disease. However, mixed groups present considerable difficulties, because these individuals often have widely differing needs. In our view, a better solution is individual therapy for these patients.

Lastly, we turn to the timing and duration of therapy. Although both of these factors may well affect the outcome of therapy, neither of them has been subjected to controlled clinical trials. Clinical experience suggests that the occasions when therapy is most commonly needed are immediately after initial diagnosis, at recurrence or when there is evidence of advancing disease, and during terminal illness. However, since individual patients will require psychological intervention at varying times depending on their particular circumstances, psychotherapy should be made available at every stage of the cancer process (Sellick and Crooks, 1999). With regard to the duration of therapy, as we have noted there are wide variations, ranging from 4 weekly sessions (Weisman et al, 1980) to weekly sessions for a whole year (Spiegel et al, 1981). The optimum number of sessions has not been determined empirically, but it is obvious that this will vary according to the individual needs of patients and the stage of the disease. In a systematic review of group treatments, Sherman et al (2004) concluded that there was evidence for the effectiveness of both brief structured interventions and longer-term interactive groups. Generally speaking, brief therapy is appropriate for patients with early cancer, whereas patients with more advanced disease will require more prolonged therapy.

Comparison of group therapies

We have previously described studies of the effect of individual and group psychological therapy on quality of life and on survival. The question arises as to which model of group therapy provides the best results. As far as survival is concerned, no studies comparing different kinds of group therapy have been reported. With regard to quality of life, a comprehensive meta-analytical study of psychological interventions (individual and group combined) revealed that such interventions significantly improved emotional adjustment and functional adjustment, as well as disease- and treatment-related symptoms, but there were no significant differences in outcome between various kinds of intervention (Meyer and Mark, 1995). However, the authors point out that their results were based on studies comparing psychological treatment with untreated controls. They recommend that studies should be conducted which directly compare different therapies.

Cunningham and Tocco (1989) compared psychoeducational group therapy, including training in coping skills, with supportive therapy that included supportive discussions, ventilation of feelings, and information sharing. The patients had various cancers, the commonest of which was breast cancer. Greater improvement in affective symptoms occurred in the group that received coping skills training than among the patients who received the supportive intervention only. Similar results were reported by Telch and Telch (1986), who compared group coping skills training with supportive group therapy and a no-treatment control in patients with various cancers who showed 'marked psychosocial distress.' Their results demonstrated consistent superiority of the coping skills intervention over supportive group therapy and the untreated control. In a small pilot study, Bottomley et al (1996) assigned newly diagnosed, psychologically distressed cancer patients to either a cognitive-behavioural group, a social support group, or a non-intervention group. Their results showed that CBT was superior to social support in improving patients' coping styles. These few studies provide some preliminary evidence which suggests that cognitive-behavioural methods may be more successful than supportive discussions in group therapy. However, such evidence is insufficient to allow firm conclusions to be drawn. A study of 353 women within 1 year of diagnosis of primary breast cancer, who were randomized to either supportive-expressive group therapy or an educational control condition, revealed no evidence of a reduction in distress associated with supportive-expressive group therapy (Classen et al, 2008).

An interesting suggestion has been put forward by Bloch and Kissane (1995), who argue that CBT may be more applicable to early-stage disease to help patients to adjust to their potential 'survivorship.' Supportive-expressive therapy, on the other hand, encourages the sharing of feelings about existential concerns, and may for that reason be more suitable for patients with metastatic disease. The evidence to date from two randomized trials lends support to Bloch and Kissane's suggestion. Whereas supportive-expressive group therapy was found to relieve emotional distress in women with metastatic breast cancer (Classen et al, 2001), no such effect was found in women with primary breast cancer (Classen et al, 2008). However, with regard to individual CBT, the randomized trials that we have conducted indicate that CBT results in a significant improvement in quality of life for patients with predominantly primary cancer (Greer et al, 1992), as well as for patients with advanced cancer (see Chapter 12).

A different approach has been recommended by a leading researcher and therapist who has personally experienced and survived cancer:

> It surely makes sense to use therapies combining all the modalities that responsible therapists have described as helping patients. There is no room for partisanship here.

> (Cunningham, 1999, p. 000)

The small number of studies that have combined supportive-expressive group therapy with CBT in women with breast cancer have not demonstrated consistently positive results (Boutin, 2007).

Summary and conclusions

1. Both individual and group psychotherapy should be made available for cancer patients who, on psychological screening, show evidence of persistent emotional distress (clinical anxiety, depression, and/or helplessness/hopelessness).

2. Group therapy conducted with cancer patients can be categorized under three headings, namely psychoeducational, supportive-expressive, and cognitive-behavioural, although there is some overlap between these models.

3. Studies that have compared the different models of group therapy are rare. Preliminary evidence suggests an advantage for CBT, but further studies are required before any firm conclusions can be drawn.

4. Homogeneous groups (i.e. patients with the same cancer and stage of disease) consisting of 6 to 12 members are recommended.

5. Therapy is most commonly required following the diagnosis of cancer, at recurrence, and during terminal illness, but should be available throughout the course of cancer.

6. The duration of therapy documented in the literature varies widely. Clinical experience suggests that patients with early-stage cancer can benefit from brief therapy, whereas more prolonged therapy is required for patients with advanced or terminal illness.

7. Studies are required to determine the comparative effectiveness of different models of group therapy, the optimum times for psychological intervention, and the optimum duration of such intervention.

Chapter 17

Concluding remarks

In this book we have tried to achieve a balance between theory, research data, and practical comment, updating the original edition in each area. However, the prevailing emphasis remains on the clinical applications of cognitive behavioural techniques to people with cancer. Despite the large quantity of work demonstrating the effectiveness of CBT for people with cancer, there are still relatively few practical texts that describe 'how to do it.' Inevitably we have not been able to cover the whole area of psychosocial oncology. We have not attempted to review all of the studies of psychological morbidity in cancer, nor have we tried to draw together the increasing body of data on coping. Instead, in Chapters 1 and 2 we have used some of the research evidence to illustrate the model of adjustment to cancer that forms the basis of APT. Chapters 3 and 4 contain reviews of the literature concerning the efficacy of cognitive behavioural interventions in cancer, and the evidence that mental adjustment may influence disease outcome. Part Two of the book has used the model described in Part One as the framework for a practical guide to psychotherapy for patients with cancer.

Although the effectiveness of APT has been demonstrated, further questions need to be answered. This includes identifying the effective components of the treatment package, determining whether (as the evidence suggests) APT is more effective than other forms of therapy, such as counselling, and ascertaining which patients are most likely to benefit from it. Perhaps most importantly, we need to find a way to disseminate the techniques that have been shown to be effective in randomized controlled trials conducted by experts to clinical situations. Work in this field is now moving in two exciting directions. First, simpler 'first-aid' methods are being disseminated to oncology professionals, and secondly, new techniques are being refined for use by CBT therapists when working with more severe and complex cases. We hope that this book will be of use to both in taking cognitive behaviour for people with cancer into its next phase of development.

Appendix 1

Coping with Cancer

Everyone learns to deal with cancer in their own individual way, bringing their unique strengths and resources to the process of coping. There are as many different reactions to cancer as there are people with the illness. Psychological therapy is about helping you to find what works best for you. This may mean exploring new ways to think about the disease and its impact on your life, trying new methods to cope with the illness, or even just getting back to some of the things you used to do before the cancer came along. How people cope seems to depend very much on how they view themselves and their illness. Disturbing thoughts and feelings, such as anger, guilt, and fear, are common: they are part of the process of coming to terms with cancer. Here are some examples of the sorts of thoughts and emotions that you might have had:

Thoughts	Emotion
Why me? I've done nothing to deserve this.	Anger
Why do I feel so tired? Has the cancer really gone?	Fear
Will people avoid me because I've got the big C?	Fear and shame
There's nothing I can do. It's hopeless.	Depression
I'm not a normal person any more.	Depression
I know that I can deal with this, with the help of my family and the doctors.	Hope

Some reactions, like the last one, can help you live life to the full and fight back against the cancer. Others, if they persist, can make it harder to cope. You probably have a mixture of the two sorts. You may think that reactions like this are 'just part of you' and cannot be changed, but, as the rest of this leaflet explains, by working on how you think and what you do it is possible to have a stronger and more comfortable way of coping.

Psychological therapy

The psychological therapy that you are starting can help you to cope better, in partnership with any physical treatments you may be having. It takes about 6 to 12 hourly sessions once a week. Your therapist will help you to identify the problems you face and your strengths and weaknesses in dealing with them. You can then decide together which problems to tackle and how best to do this. If you have a partner, you may choose for him or her to come to some of the sessions: some of the problems you have may best be overcome by the two of you working together.

Some of the methods used are set out below. Some will be helpful to you, others may not. You and your therapist will decide which to try, and you will learn how and when to use them. As you read about them, think about whether they could be useful to you. With what sort of problems might they be helpful?

Problem solving

You are probably already a very good problem solver, but cancer can make you feel paralysed. Once you have identified the problems you want to work on, you can think of possible solutions with the help of your therapist. Your partner can make a contribution to your coping, and you will have another set of ideas on what to do. You will learn to decide which solution to try first, and then be helped to put it into practice.

For instance, many people feel tongue-tied when seeing their doctor and forget all the important questions they want to ask. Other patients who have used the therapy have come up with a number of solutions using problem solving with their therapist or partner:

1. Write down what you want to ask, and read it out.
2. Bring someone with you to the consultation.
3. Rehearse what you want to say with your therapist or partner.

You can probably think of more. Therapy is about enabling you to recover your confidence to be an effective problem solver.

Expressing feelings

You may well have strong, unpleasant feelings such as fear, sadness, or anger. You may not want to burden other people with them or feel unsafe expressing them, but research suggests that being open about how you feel can help you to cope better. You will have the chance to talk about such feelings with your therapist and to improve communication with important people in your life so that you can support each other better.

Dealing with negative thoughts

When coping with cancer, you may face very unpleasant experiences, major changes in your way of life, and uncertainty about the future. When you think about these things, some of your thoughts will help you cope, whereas others may be unhelpful and lead to distress. Once you have faced your negative emotions and shared them with your therapist, you can start to explore the thoughts behind them. Some examples of thoughts which make it more difficult to cope are:

'I know I'm going to die from the cancer.'
'There's no point in doing anything.'
'No one will love me if my hair falls out.'
'I can't cope.'

Such thoughts can lead you to underestimate your coping abilities and overestimate your problems; we call them negative automatic thoughts because they are unrealistically pessimistic and because they seem to come from nowhere and 'automatically' pop into your mind. In therapy you will learn to separate realistic negative thoughts from extreme or unhelpful negative thoughts. They are difficult to spot to start with (you are probably not aware that you have them), and the first step is to learn to recognize them. You can keep a diary of when you get these thoughts, what might have triggered them, and what you feel and do when they come into your mind. Many people find that just catching the thoughts allows them to get more control over them, but if you are feeling very anxious or depressed this may not work in itself. You may need more help from the therapist to change the patterns of self-defeating thinking. You can start to ask yourself questions to examine how realistic or helpful these negative thoughts really are, and start to find alternative, more constructive ways to think. Research has shown that doing this can improve your mood and make you feel more in control of your situation. Here is an example of how this works:

A man with cancer felt a twinge in his hip. He immediately thought 'I've got cancer in my bones.' This is a negative automatic thought—he had jumped to the worst possible conclusion. Not surprisingly, he felt anxious. He questioned his reason for believing this and remembered that he had had this pain on and off for years, long before he got cancer. He was able to challenge the thought with the reply: 'I had arthritis in my hip long before I got cancer. The last check-up showed the cancer hadn't spread. These are just ordinary aches and pains.' This reduced the belief that the cancer had spread, and so he felt less anxious.

Do not worry if this seems complicated. If you and your therapist decide to use this technique, you will learn it gradually, using examples from your own negative thoughts.

Improving the quality of life

The goal of all our therapy is to improve the quality of your life. When you have cancer, you may miss out on some of things you enjoy. This may be because of physical ill health, because you spend a lot of time thinking about your illness and its treatment, or because you do not see the point in going on with ordinary life. You can reduce the effect the illness has on you and fight back by doing things you enjoy and things which give you a sense of achievement. We have found that this gives people back a feeling of being in control of their lives. It also makes them feel connected with the real world, so they are a person in their own right and not just a 'cancer patient.' Your therapist may help you to keep a diary of what you are doing that is pleasurable or that gives you a feeling of achievement. You can build on this by planning challenging and enjoyable activities into your week. It is important to set your expectations at the right level—if you are tired and weak, making a cup of tea may be a major achievement in itself. If you are unable to do everything as before, do not give up: do what you can, and above all give yourself credit for it. You and your therapist will discuss ways to use your time and energy to best advantage.

Learning new coping methods

There are several other coping methods as well as the ones we have already mentioned. Depending on your problems, your therapist may suggest other techniques. Many people find practising relaxation helpful. Physical tension and distress can build up in a vicious circle where each increases the other. You and your therapist may decide to try to break the circle with relaxation exercises. You will learn them either from a tape or CD, or from your therapist, and practise them regularly. Being able to relax may help you to deal with stressful situations.

Conclusions

You may be coping very well already, but have a few problems or worries, or you may be in great difficulties and doubt that you will ever overcome them. Whatever your situation, you and your therapist can work together alongside your other treatments to help you to cope with cancer and to ensure that you are still in control of your life.

You may find it helpful to read this leaflet again now, picking up the points that you think apply to you and any with which you disagree. Your therapist will be happy to talk about any questions or concerns you may have about this therapy and how you can use it.

Tick a box if you think one of these could be helpful to you:

Problem solving	☐
Expressing feelings	☐
Dealing with negative thoughts	☐
Improving your quality of life	☐
Learning new coping methods	☐

Would you be willing to practise self-help assignments between sessions?

I am willing to practise self help
assignments between sessions ☐

Appendix 2

Thinking Errors

When people feel overwhelmed or demoralized they often get things out of proportion. This can lead them to exaggerate the real problems they are facing, and to underestimate their ability to cope with these problems. In these situations a person's thinking shows certain 'negative distortions' or 'thinking errors.' Some of the examples below may help you to recognize the distortions in your negative thoughts.

1. Overgeneralization

This distortion means that you see a single negative event as a never-ending pattern of defeat. For instance, if you have a row with your partner the day after you get back from hospital, you think 'It's the cancer. We'll always be arguing, things will never be the same again. We might as well split up now and get it over with.'

2. Magnification and minimization

You exaggerate the importance of some things, such as other patients' strengths and coping abilities, while at the same time playing down others until they appear insignificant, such as your own methods of coping. You may say to yourself 'Everyone is coping better than me. I'm just a heap.'

3. All-or-nothing thinking

The world is seen in absolute, black-and-white terms. If your performance falls short of perfect you see yourself as a complete failure, or if the treatment is not 100% likely to be successful you see it as useless.

For example, a man who had been told that he could not be cured of cancer said 'If I can't be cured, there's no point in doing anything. I might as well die now.' Yet with appropriate treatment he could have months or years of active life.

4. Selective attention

If you feel depressed you are only able to think about the negative parts of your life. You selectively attend to these while ignoring all the positive things that are happening to you.

For example, a woman with breast cancer who was about to receive chemo-therapy could only think of the side-effects that she would experience over the course of treatment. She thought of the unpleasantness of the next few months and ignored the fact that if the treatment was successful she would be able to enjoy the rest of her life. By focusing on this she also failed to see what she was able to do and to enjoy on a day-to-day basis.

5. Negative predictions

The future for many people with cancer is uncertain. But you can turn this into a negative certainty by assuming the worst:

'I know this treatment won't work.'
'I won't be able to cope if the cancer comes back.'
'If I lose my hair as a result of this treatment, my partner will no longer find me attractive.'
'Even if I'm cured of cancer I know something else will come along to cause problems for me.'

6. Mind-reading

Instead of finding out what people are thinking you jump to conclusions, but attempts to read other people's minds are rarely successful.

For example, a patient who had been successfully treated for cancer of the salivary gland felt herself to be under great stress at home. She thought that her family were deliberately not helping her because they were lazy and didn't care about her. In fact, they had wrongly assumed that once she was physically well everything could get back to normal immediately. They were acting out of ignorance, not malice.

7. Shoulds and oughts

You try to motivate yourself with 'shoulds' and 'oughts', but end up feeling guilty. For example, 'I should be able to do everything I did before I got cancer. Even though I don't feel well, I should still be looking after my children.'

When you direct 'should' statements towards others or life in general you feel anger and resentment:

'My husband and daughter should know I'm under stress and treat me differently.'
'I have tried to live a good life, I shouldn't have got cancer.'

8. Labelling

You apply a critical label to yourself instead of accurately describing the situation. Instead of saying 'I didn't do that job as well as I might have done', you say to yourself 'I'm a failure.' Or if you find it difficult to concentrate because of the stress you are under, you say 'I'm an idiot.'

9. Personalization

You see yourself as the cause of some negative event for which you are not necessarily responsible. If your children are badly behaved, you say to yourself 'It must be my fault.' If friends cancel a visit, you say 'It must be because I have cancer.'

Identifying negative thoughts is the first step in learning to change your thinking. Real negative events can be exaggerated and distorted until they seem to be enormous problems which you cannot hope to solve. If you master the thinking errors you can cut your problems down to size, and devote your energy to solving them rather than just worrying about them.

Weekly Activity Schedule

Time	Monday	Tuesday	Wednesday	Thursday	Friday	Saturday	Sunday
9–10							
10–11							
11–12							
12–1							
1–2							
2–3							
3–4							
4–5							
5–6							
6–7							
7–8							
8–12							

Appendix 4

Thought Record

Situation	Physical sensations (rate from 0–10)	Emotions (rate from 0–10)	Automatic thoughts	Alternative response	Action plan

Mental Adjustment to Cancer (MACS) Scale

Name: _____ Date: _____

A number of statements are given below which describe people's reactions to having cancer. Please circle the appropriate number to the right of each statement, indicating how far it applies to you at present. For example, if the statement definitely does *not* apply to you, then you should circle 1 in the first column.

	Definitely does *not* apply to me	Does *not* apply to me	Applies to me	Definitely applies to me
1. I have been doing things that I believe will improve my health (e.g. I have changed my diet)	1	2	3	4
2. I feel I can't do anything to cheer myself up	1	2	3	4
3. I feel that problems with my health prevent me from planning ahead	1	2	3	4
4. I believe that my positive attitude will benefit my health	1	2	3	4
5. I don't dwell on my illness	1	2	3	4
6. I firmly believe that I will get better	1	2	3	4
7. I feel that nothing I can do will make any difference	1	2	3	4
8. I've left it all to my doctors	1	2	3	4
9. I feel that life is hopeless	1	2	3	4
10. I have been doing things that I believe will improve my health (e.g. exercise)	1	2	3	4

(Continued)

	Definitely does *not* apply to me	Does *not* apply to me	Applies to me	Definitely applies to me
11. Since my cancer diagnosis I now realize how precious life is, and I'm making the most of it	1	2	3	4
12. I've put myself in the hands of God	1	2	3	4
13. I have plans for the future (e.g. holiday, jobs, housing)	1	2	3	4
14. I worry about the cancer returning or getting worse	1	2	3	4
15. I've had a good life — what's left is a bonus	1	2	3	4
16. I think my state of mind can make a lot of difference to my health	1	2	3	4
17. I feel that there is nothing I can do to help myself	1	2	3	4
18. I try to carry on my life as I've always done	1	2	3	3
19. I would like to make contact with others in the same boat				
20. I am determined to put it all behind me	1	2	3	4
21. I have difficulty in believing that this has happened to me	1	2	3	4
22. I suffer great anxiety about it	1	2	3	4
23. I am not very hopeful about the future	1	2	3	4
24. At the moment I take one day at a time	1	2	3	4
25. I feel like giving up	1	2	3	4
26. I try to keep a sense of humour about it	1	2	3	4
27. Other people worry about me more than I do	1	2	3	4
28. I think of other people who are worse off	1	2	3	4

	Definitely does *not* apply to me	Does *not* apply to me	Applies to me	Definitely applies to me
29. I am trying to get as much information as I can about cancer	1	2	3	4
30. I feel that I can't control what is happening	1	2	3	4
31. I try to have a very positive attitude	1	2	3	4
32. I keep quite busy, so I don't have time to think about it	1	2	3	4
33. I avoid finding out more about it	1	2	3	4
34. I see my illness as a challenge	1	2	3	4
35. I feel fatalistic about it	1	2	3	4
36. I feel completely at a loss about what to do	1	2	3	4
37. I feel very angry about what has happened to me	1	2	3	4
38. I don't really believe I have cancer	1	2	3	4
39. I count my blessings	1	2	3	4
40. I try to fight the illness	1	2	3	4

(Watson and Greer, 1988)

Cancer Coping Questionnaire (21-item version)

Name.............................   Hospital number........................

People have many ways of coping with the stress that cancer puts them under. How stressful has the last week been for you?

Very stressful   Moderately stressful   Slightly stressful   Not at all stressful

☐   ☐   ☐   ☐

Have you worried about cancer in the last week?

Most of the time   A lot of the time   Some of the time   None of the time

☐   ☐   ☐   ☐

On the following pages there is a list of different methods of coping. Think about how you have coped with your illness in the *last week*, and circle how often you have used each method described. No one uses all the ways of coping described, but everyone uses some of them.

In the last week did you:

		Very often	Often	Sometimes	Not at all
1.	Make definite plans for the future?	4	3	2	1
2.	Try breathing slowly and deeply to cope with anxiety?	4	3	2	1
3.	Distract yourself from worrying thoughts?	4	3	2	1
4.	Remind yourself that aches and pains could be caused by things other than the cancer spreading?	4	3	2	1
5.	Make a list of priorities for the week so that you got important things done?	4	3	2	1
6.	Stand back to get the seriousness of your illness into proportion?	4	3	2	1

	Very often	Often	Sometimes	Not at all
7. Look for what strengths you have to cope with cancer?	4	3	2	1
8. Cope with frustration by channelling it into other things (e.g. physical activity like housework or gardening)?	4	3	2	1
9. Remind yourself of what things you still have in life despite cancer?	4	3	2	1
10. Organize your day so that you got the most out of it, despite cancer?	4	3	2	1
11. Practise relaxation?	4	3	2	1
12. Answer back worrying thoughts?	4	3	2	1
13. Plan your day so that you got on with some activities unrelated to cancer?	4	3	2	1
14. Make sure you thought of some of the positive aspects of your life?	4	3	2	1

If you are in a close relationship, think of how you and your partner have coped in the last week.

In the last week did you:

	Very often	Often	Sometimes	Not at all
15. Involve your partner in an activity that helped you cope with cancer?	4	3	2	1
16. Talk with your partner about the impact of cancer on your lives?	4	3	2	1
17. Ask your partner what (s)he was thinking, rather than making assumptions?	4	3	2	1
18. Try to see cancer as a challenge that you and your partner have to face together?	4	3	2	1
19. Discuss how your partner could help support you?	4	3	2	1
20. Talk to your partner about how you could organize things to take some pressure off you (e.g. changing who does household chores)?	4	3	2	1
21. Think of how cancer had brought you and your partner closer together?	4	3	2	1

Cancer Concerns Checklist

We would like to know the different concerns that may have been worrying you about your illness and treatment over the <u>last few weeks</u>. Please remember to answer all the questions.

Tick only one box in each section

The illness itself (what is it, is it better, etc.)

- Not a worry
- Slightly worried
- Moderately worried
- Very worried
- Extremely worried

Treatment for the illness

- Not a worry
- Slightly worried
- Moderately worried
- Very worried
- Extremely worried

How I have been feeling physically

- Not a worry
- Slightly worried
- Moderately worried
- Very worried
- Extremely worried

Not being able to do things

- Not a worry
- Slightly worried
- Moderately worried
- Very worried
- Extremely worried

My job

- Not a worry
- Slightly worried
- Moderately worried
- Very worried
- Extremely worried

Finances

- Not a worry
- Slightly worried
- Moderately worried
- Very worried
- Extremely worried

Feeling upset or distressed

- Not a worry
- Slightly worried
- Moderately worried
- Very worried
- Extremely worried

Feeling different from other people

- Not a worry
- Slightly worried
- Moderately worried
- Very worried
- Extremely worried

How I feel about myself as a man or woman

- Not a worry
- Slightly worried
- Moderately worried
- Very worried
- Extremely worried

My relationship with my partner

- Not a worry
- Slightly worried
- Moderately worried
- Very worried
- Extremely worried

My relationship with others

- Not a worry
- Slightly worried
- Moderately worried
- Very worried
- Extremely worried

The support I have

- Not a worry
- Slightly worried
- Moderately worried
- Very worried
- Extremely worried

The future

- Not a worry
- Slightly worried
- Moderately worried
- Very worried
- Extremely worried

Any other concern? Please describe

- Not a worry
- Slightly worried
- Moderately worried
- Very worried
- Extremely worried

References

Aapro MS, Molassiotis A and Oliver I (2005) Anticipatory nausea and vomiting. *Supportive Care in Cancer*, **13**, 117–21.

Ahmedzai SH and Shrivastav SP (2000) Breathlessness. *Medicine*, **28**, 12–15.

Aitken-Swan J and Easson EC (1959) Reactions of cancer patients on being told their diagnosis. *British Medical Journal*, **1**, 779–83.

Akechi T *et al* (2008) Psychotherapy for depression among incurable cancer patients. *Cochrane Database of Systematic Reviews* 2: CD005537 75.

Aldridge D (1992) The needs of individual patients in clinical research. *Advances*, **8**, 58–65.

Allison PJ, Guichard C and Gilain L (2000) A prospective investigation of dispositional optimism as a predictor of health-related quality of life in head and neck cancer patients. *Quality of Life Research*, **9**, 951–60.

Andersen BL (1986) Sexual difficulties for women following cancer treatment. In: Andersen BL, ed. *Women with Cancer*, pp. 257–88. New York: Springer.

Andersen BL, Yan H-C and Farrar WB (2008) Psychologic intervention improves survival for breast cancer patients. *Cancer*, **113**, 3450–58.

Andrykowski MA, Brady MJ and Henslee-Downey PJ (1994) Psychosocial factors predictive of survival after allogeneic bone marrow transplantation. *Psychosomatic Medicine*, **56**, 432–39.

Angell M (1985) Disease as a reflection of the psyche. *New England Journal of Medicine*, **312**, 1570–72.

Antiemetic Subcommittee of the Multinational Association of Supportive Care in Cancer (MASCC) (1998) Prevention of chemotherapy- and radiotherapy-induced emesis: results of Perugia Consensus Conference. *Annals of Oncology*, **9**, 811–19.

Antoni MH and Goodkin K (1988) Host moderator variables in the promotion of cervical neoplasia. I. Personality facets. *Journal of Psychosomatic Research*, **32**, 327–38.

Antoni MH *et al* (2001) Cognitive-behavioural stress management intervention decreases the prevalence of depression and enhances benefit finding among women under treatment for early-stage breast cancer. *Health Psychology*, **20**, 20–32.

Antoni MH *et al* (2006) Reduction of cancer-specific thought intrusions and anxiety symptoms with a stress management intervention among women undergoing treatment for breast cancer. *American Journal of Psychiatry*, **163**, 1791–97.

Armes J *et al* (2007) A randomized controlled trial to evaluate the effectiveness of a brief, behaviorally oriented intervention for cancer-related fatigue. *Cancer*, **110**, 1385–95.

Badger TA, Braden CJ, Longman AJ and Mishel MM (1999) Depression burden, self-help interventions, and social support in women receiving treatment for breast cancer. *Journal of Psychosocial Oncology*, **17**, 17–35.

Baider L, Cooper CL and De-Nour AK, eds (1996) *Cancer and the Family*. Chichester: John Wiley & Sons Ltd.

Bartlett FC (1932) *Remembering*. Cambridge: Cambridge University Press.

Bartley T (2011) Cancer: psychological implications. In: *Mindfulness-Based Cognitive Therapy for Cancer: gently turning towards*. London: Wiley-Blackwell.

Barton RT (1965) Life after laryngectomy. *Laryngoscope*, **75**, 1408–15.

Beck AT (1976) *Cognitive Therapy and the Emotional Disorders*. London: Penguin.

Beck AT (1988) *Love is Never Enough*. New York: Harper Row.

Beck AT *et al* (1961) An inventory for measuring depression. *Archives of General Psychiatry*, **4**, 561–71.

Beck AT, Rush AJ, Shaw BF and Emery G (1979) *Cognitive Therapy of Depression*. New York: Guilford Press.

Beck JS (1995) *Cognitive Therapy: basics and beyond*. New York: Guilford Press.

Beck R and Fernandez E (1998) Cognitive-behavioral therapy in the treatment of anger: a meta-analysis. *Cognitive Therapy and Research*, **22**, 63–74.

Beltman MW, Oude Voshaar RC and Speckens AE (2010) Cognitive-behavioural therapy for depression in people with a somatic disease: meta-analysis of randomised controlled trials. *British Journal of Psychiatry*, **197**, 11–19.

Bennett-Levy J *et al*, eds (2004) *Oxford Guide to Behavioural Experiments in Cognitive Therapy*. Oxford: Oxford University Press.

Berger AM (2009) Update on the state of the science: sleep-wake disturbances in adult patients with cancer. *Oncology Nursing Forum*, **36**, 165–77.

Berglund G, Bolund C, Gustaffson O and Sjoden P (1994) A randomized study of a rehabilitation program for cancer patients: the 'starting again' group. *Psycho-Oncology*, **3**, 109–20.

Bloch S and Kissane DW (1995) Psychological care and breast cancer. *Lancet*, **346**, 1114.

Bloom JR (1986) Social support and adjustment to breast cancer. In: Andersen BL, ed. *Women with Cancer*, pp. 204–29. New York: Springer.

Bloom JR and Spiegel D (1984) The relationship of two dimensions of social support to the psychological well-being and social functioning of women with advanced breast cancer. *Social Science and Medicine*, **19**, 831–7.

Boelan PA, de Keijser J, van den Hout MA and van den Bout J (2007) Treatment of complicated grief: a comparison between cognitive behaviour therapy and supportive counselling. *Journal of Consulting and Clinical Psychology*, **75**, 271–84.

Boesen E *et al* (2005) Psychoeducational intervention for patients with cutaneous malignant melanoma: a replication study. *Journal of Clinical Oncology*, **23**, 1270–77.

Bohart A (1980) Toward a cognitive theory of catharsis. *Psychotherapy: Theory, Research and Practice*, **17**, 192–201.

Bohart A, Elliott R, Greenberg LS and Watson JC (2002) Empathy. In: Norcross JC, ed. *Psychotherapy Relationships that Work*, pp. 89–108. New York: Oxford University Press.

Borkovec TD (1994) The nature, functions, and origins of worry. In: Davey GCL and Tallis F, eds. *Worrying: perspectives on theory, assessment and treatment*, pp. 5–34. New York: John Wiley & Sons Ltd.

Borkovec TD and Hennings BC (1978) The role of physiological attention-focusing in the relaxation treatment of sleep disturbance, general tension, and specific stress reaction. *Behaviour Research and Therapy*, **16**, 17–19.

Borysenko J *et al* (1986) *Beth Israel Hospital: Mind/Body Group Program Handbook* (unpublished manuscript).

Bottomley A *et al* (1996) A pilot study of cognitive-behavioural therapy and social support group interventions with newly diagnosed cancer patients. *Journal of Psychosocial Oncology*, **14**, 65–83.

Boutin DL (2007) Effectiveness of cognitive behavioral and supportive-expressive group therapy for women diagnosed with breast cancer: a review of the literature. *Journal for Specialists in Group Work*, **32**, 267–84.

Bovbjerg DH (2006) The continuing problem of post chemotherapy nausea and vomiting: contributions of classical conditioning. *Autonomic Neuroscience: Basic and Clinical*, **129**, 92–8.

Bradford Hill A (1961) *Principles of Medical Statistics*. London: The Lancet Ltd.

Brady SS and Helgeson VS (1999) Social support and adjustment to recurrence of breast cancer. *Journal of Psychosocial Oncology*, **17**, 37–55.

Breitbart W and Cohen KR (1998) Delirium. In: Holland JC, ed. *Psycho-Oncology*, pp. 564–75. New York: Oxford University Press.

Brewin CR *et al* (1998) Intrusive memories and depression in cancer patients. *Behaviour Research and Therapy*, **36**, 1131–42.

Bruera E, Miller L and McCallion S (1990) Cognitive failure in patients with terminal cancer: a prospective longitudinal study. *Psychosocial Aspects of Cancer*, **9**, 308–10.

Buddeberg C, Wolf C and Sieber M (1991) Coping strategies and course of disease of breast cancer patients. *Psychotherapy and Psychosomatics*, **55**, 151–7.

Bukberg J, Penman G and Holland JC (1984) Depression in hospitalised cancer patients. *Psychosomatic Medicine*, **46**, 199–212.

Burgess C *et al* (2005) Depression and anxiety in women with early breast cancer: five-year observational cohort study. *British Medical Journal*, **330**, 702–7.

Burns DD (1980) *Feeling Good: the new mood therapy*. New York: William Morrow.

Burns DD and Auerbach A (1996) Therapeutic empathy in cognitive behaviour therapy: does it really make a difference? In: Salkovskis PM, ed. *Frontiers of Cognitive Therapy*. New York: Guilford Press.

Byma EA, Given BA and Given CW (2009) The effects of mastery on pain and fatigue resolution. *Oncology Nursing Forum*, **36**, 544–52.

Cain EN *et al* (1986) Psychosocial benefits of a cancer support group. *Cancer*, **57**, 183–9.

Carter RE, Carter CA and Prosen HA (1993) Emotional and personality types of breast cancer patients and spouses. *American Journal of Family Therapy*, **20**, 300–309.

Carver CS *et al* (1993) How coping mediates the effect of optimism on distress: a study of women with early stage breast cancer. *Journal of Personality and Social Psychology*, **65**, 375–90.

Cassileth BR *et al* (1985) Psychological correlates of survival in advanced malignant disease. *New England Journal of Medicine*, **312**, 1551–5.

Castonguay LG *et al* (1996) Predicting the effect of cognitive therapy for depression: a study of unique and common factors. *Journal of Consulting and Clinical Psychology*, **64**, 497–504.

Cawley RH (1983) The principles of treatment and therapeutic evaluation. In: Shepherd M and Zangwill O, eds. *General Psychopathology*, pp. 221–43. Cambridge: Cambridge University Press.

Chemtob CM, Novaco RW, Hamada RS and Gross DM (1997) Cognitive-behavioral treatment for severe anger in posttraumatic stress disorder. *Journal of Consulting and Clinical Psychology*, **65**, 184–9.

Crichton P and Moorey S (2002) Treating pain in cancer patients. In: Turk DC and Gatchel RJ, eds. *Psychological Approaches to Pain Management: a practitioner's handbook*, 2nd edn. New York: Guilford Press.

Clark DA and Steer RA (1996) Empirical status of the cognitive model of anxiety and depression. In: Salkovskis PM, ed. *Frontiers of Cognitive Therapy*. New York: Guilford Press.

Classen C, Koopman C, Angell K and Spiegel D (1996) Coping styles associated with psychological adjustment to advanced breast cancer. *Health Psychology*, **15**, 434–7.

Classen C, Sephton SE, Diamond S and Spiegel D (1998) Studies of life-extending psychosocial interventions. In: Holland JC, ed. *Psycho-Oncology*, pp. 730–42. New York: Oxford University Press.

Classen C *et al* (2001) Supportive expressive group therapy and distress in patients with metastatic breast cancer: a randomized clinical intervention. *Archives of General Psychiatry*, **58**, 494–501.

Classen CC, Kraemer HC and Blasey C (2008) Supportive expressive group therapy for primary breast cancer: a randomized prospective multicenter trial. *Psycho-Oncology*, **17**, 438–47.

Cochran D, Hacker NF, Wellisch DK and Berek JS (1987) Sexual functioning after treatment for endometrial cancer. *Journal of Psychosocial Oncology*, **5**, 47–61.

Cohn KH (1982) Chemotherapy from an insider's perspective. *Lancet*, **i**, 1006–9.

Cooper A (1982) Disabilities and how to live with them: Hodgkin's disease. *Lancet*, **i**, 612–13.

Cormie PJ, Nairn M and Welsh J (2008) Control of pain in adults with cancer: summary of SIGN guidelines. *British Medical Journal*, **337**, a2154.

Cort E *et al* (2009) Palliative care nurses' experiences of training in cognitive behaviour therapy and taking part in a randomized controlled trial. *International Journal of Palliative Nursing*, **15**, 290–98.

Coursey K, Dawson JJ and Luce JK (1975) Comparative anxiety levels of cancer patients and family members. *Proceedings of the American Association for Cancer Research*, **16**, 246.

Cox DR (1972) Regression models and life tables. *Journal of the Royal Statistical Society*, **34B**, 187–202.

Coyne JC and Palmer SC (2007) Does psychotherapy extend survival? Some methodological problems overlooked. *Journal of Clinical Oncology*, **25**, 4852–53.

Coyne JC, Lepore SJ and Palmer SC (2006) Efficacy of psychosocial interventions in cancer care: evidence is weaker than it first looks. *Annals of Behavioral Medicine*, **32**, 104–10.

Coyne JC, Thomas B and Stefanek M (2009) Time to let go of the illusion that psychotherapy extends the survival of cancer patients: reply to Kraemer, Kuchler and Spiegel (2009). *Psychological Bulletin*, **135**, 179–82.

Crary WG and Crary GC (1974) Emotional crisis and cancer. *Cancer*, **24**, 36–9.

Cunningham AJ (1995) Adjuvant psychological therapy for cancer patients: putting it on the same footing as adjunctive medical therapies. *Psycho-Oncology*, **9**, 367–71.

Cunningham AJ (1999) Mind-body research in psychooncology: what directions will be most useful? *Advances in Mind-Body Medicine*, **15**, 252–5.

Cunningham AJ and Tocco EK (1989) A randomized trial of group psychoeducational therapy for cancer patients. *Patient Education and Counseling*, **14**, 101–14.

Cunningham AJ, Lockwood GA and Cunningham JA (1991) A relationship between self-efficacy and quality of life in cancer patients. *Patient Education and Counselling*, **17**, 71–8.

Cunningham AJ, Lockwood GA and Edmonds CV (1993) Which cancer patients benefit from a brief, group, coping skills programme? *International Journal of Psychiatry in Medicine*, **23**, 383–98.

Cunningham AJ, Edmonds CVI, Jenkins G and Lockwood GA (1995) A randomised comparison of two forms of brief, group, psychoeducational program for cancer patients: weekly sessions vs a 'weekend intensive.' *International Journal of Psychiatry in Medicine*, **25**, 171–87.

Cunningham AJ *et al* (1998) A randomised controlled trial of the effects of group psychological therapy on survival in women with metastatic breast cancer. *Psycho-Oncology*, **7**, 508–17.

Currier J, Holland J, Coleman R and Neimeyer RA (2006) Bereavement following violent death: an assault on life and meaning. In: Stevenson R and Cox G, eds. *Perspectives on Violence and Violent Death*, pp. 175–200. Amityville, NY: Baywood.

Dalton JA, Feuerstein M, Carlson J and Roghman K (1994) Biobehavioral pain profile: development and psychometric properties. *Pain*, **57**, 95–107.

Dalton JA, Keefe FJ, Carlson J and Youngblood R (2004) Tailoring cognitive-behavioral treatment for cancer pain. *Pain Management Nursing*, **5**, 3–18.

Dana CM *et al* (2009) Psychosocial interventions for adolescent cancer patients: a systematic review of the literature. *Psycho-Oncology*, **18**, 683–90.

Dattilio FM (1997) Family therapy. In: Leahy RL, ed. *Practising Cognitive Therapy: a guide to interventions*, pp. 409–50. Northvale, NJ: Jason Aronson.

Dattilio FM and Padesky CA (1990) *Cognitive Therapy with Couples*. Saratosa, FL: Professional Resource Exchange.

Davidson JR, MacLean AW, Brundage MD and Schulze K (2002) Sleep disturbance in cancer patients. *Social Science and Medicine*, **54**, 1309–21.

Dean C and Surtees PG (1995) Do psychological factors predict survival in breast cancer? *Journal of Psychosomatic Research*, **13**, 47–66.

Deffenbacher JL (1999) Cognitive-behavioral conceptualization and treatment of anger. *Journal of Clinical Psychology*, **55**, 295–309.

de Haes JCJM *et al* (1987). Evaluation of the quality of life of patients with advanced ovarian cancer treated with combination chemotherapy. In: Aaronson NK and Beckmann J, eds. *The Quality of Life of Cancer Patients*, pp. 215–26. New York: Raven Press.

Derogatis LR (1983) *Psychosocial Adjustment to Illness Scale (PAIS and PAIS–SR). Scoring, procedures and administration manual I*. Baltimore, MD: Clinical Psychometric Research.

Derogatis LR, Abeloff MD and Melisaratos N (1979) Psychological coping mechanisms and survival time in metastatic breast cancer. *Journal of the American Medical Association*, **249**, 751–7.

Devlin HB, Plant JA and Griffin M (1971) Aftermath of surgery for ano-rectal cancer. *British Medical Journal*, **3**, 413–18.

Di Clemente KJ and Temoshok L (1985) Psychological adjustment to having cutaneous malignant melanoma as a predictor of follow-up clinical status. *Psychosomatic Medicine*, **47**, 81.

DiGiuseppe R and Tafrate R (2003) Anger treatment for adults: a meta-analytic review. *Clinical Psychology: Science and Practice*, **10**, 70–84.

Doorenbos A *et al* (2005) Reducing symptom limitations: a cognitive behavioural intervention randomized trial. *Psycho-Oncology*, **14**, 574–84.

Drummond S (1967). Vocal rehabilitation after laryngectomy. *British Journal of Disorders of Communication*, **2**, 39–44.

Dugas MJ and Robichaud M (2007) *Cognitive Behavioural Treatment for Generalized Anxiety Disorder*. London: Routledge.

Eardley A *et al* (1976) Colostomy: the consequences of surgery. *Clinical Oncology*, **2**, 277–83.

Edelman S, Lemon J, Bell DR and Kidman AD (1999a) Effects of group CBT on the survival time of patients with metastatic breast cancer. *Psycho-Oncology*, **8**, 474–81.

Edelman S, Bell DR and Kidman AD (1999b) A group cognitive-behaviour therapy programme with metastatic breast cancer patients. *Psycho-Oncology*, **8**, 295–305.

Edgar L, Rosberger Z and Nowlis D (1992) Coping with cancer during the first year after diagnosis. Assessment and intervention. *Cancer*, **69**, 817–28.

Edmonds CVI, Lockwood GA and Cunningham AJ (1999) Psychological response to long-term group therapy: a randomized trial with metastatic breast cancer patients. *Psycho-Oncology*, **8**, 74–91.

Eissler K R (1955) *The Psychiatrist and the Dying Patient*. New York: International University Press.

Ell K, Nishimoto R and Morvay T (1989) A longitudinal analysis of psychological adaptation among survivors of cancer. *Cancer*, **63**, 406–13.

Elliotson J (1848) *Cure of True Cancer with Mesmerism*. London: Walton and Mitchell.

Elsesser K *et al* (1994) The effects of anxiety management training on psychological variables and immune parameters in cancer patients: a pilot study. *Behavioural and Cognitive Psychotherapy*, **22**, 13–23.

Espie CA *et al* (2008) Randomised controlled clinical effectiveness trial of cognitive behavior therapy compared with treatment as usual for persistent insomnia in patients with cancer. *Journal of Clinical Oncology*, 26, 4651–8.

Evans RL and Connis RT (1995) Comparison of brief group therapies for depressed cancer patients receiving radiation treatment. *Public Health Reports*, **110**, 306–11.

Fallowfield LJ, Baum M and Maguire GP (1986) Effects of breast conservation on psychological morbidity associated with diagnosis and treatment of early breast cancer. *British Medical Journal*, **293**, 1331–4.

Faulkner A, Webb P and Maguire P (1991) Communication and counseling skills: educating health professionals working in cancer and palliative care. *Patient Education and Counseling*, **18**, 3–7.

Fawzy FI (1994) The benefits of a short-term group intervention for cancer patients. *Advances*, **10**, 17–19.

Fawzy FI and Fawzy NW (1994) A structured psychosocial intervention for cancer patients. *General Hospital Psychiatry*, **16**, 149–92.

Fawzy FI *et al* (1990a) A structured psychiatric intervention for cancer patients. I. Changes over times in methods of coping and affective disturbance. *Archives of General Psychiatry*, **47**, 720–25.

Fawzy FI *et al* (1990b) A structured psychiatric intervention for cancer patients. II. Changes over time in immunological measures. *Archives of General Psychiatry*, **47**, 729–35.

Fawzy FI *et al* (1993) Malignant melanoma: effects of an early structured psychiatric intervention, coping, and affective state on recurrence and survival 6 years later. *Archives of General Psychiatry*, **50**, 681–9.

Fawzy FI, Fawzy NW and Wheeler JG (1996) A post-hoc comparison of the efficiency of a psychoeducational intervention for melanoma patients delivered in group versus individual formats: an analysis of data from two studies. *Psycho-Oncology*, **5**, 81–9.

Feigin R *et al* (2000) The psychosocial experience of women treated for breast cancer by high-dose chemotherapy supported by autologous stem-cell transplant: a qualitative analysis of support groups. *Psycho-Oncology*, **9**, 57–68.

Feinstein AD (1983) Psychological interventions in the treatment of cancer. *Clinical Psychology Review*, **3**, 1–14.

Fennell MJV and Teasdale JD (1987) Cognitive therapy for depression: individual differences and the process of change. *Cognitive Therapy and Research*, **11**, 253–71.

Fennell MJV, Teasdale JD, Jones S and Damlé A (1987) Distraction in neurotic and endogenous depression: an investigation of negative thinking in major depressive disorders. *Psychological Medicine*, **17**, 441–52.

Fernandez-Ballesteros R, Ruiz MA and Garde S (1998) Emotional expression in healthy women and those with breast cancer. *British Journal of Health Psychology*, **3**, 41–50.

Fernandez-Marcos A *et al* (1996) Acute and anticipatory emesis in breast cancer patients. *Supportive Care in Cancer*, **4**, 370–7.

Fichten KS (1986) Self, other and situation-referant automatic thoughts: interaction between people who have a physical disability and those who do not. *Cognitive Therapy and Research*, **10**, 571–87.

Figueroa-Moseley C *et al* (2007) Behavioral interventions in treating anticipatory nausea and vomiting. *Journal of the National Comprehensive Cancer Network*, **5**, 44–50.

Finlay IG (2000) Palliative care: an introduction. *Medicine*, **28**, 1.

Fiore N (1979) Fighting cancer – one patient's perspective. *New England Journal of Medicine*, **300**, 284–9.

Fiore NA (1984) *The Road Back to Health*. New York: Bantam Books.

Fledderus M, Bohlmeijer ET and Pieterse ME (2010) Does experiential avoidance mediate the effects of maladaptive coping styles on psychopathology and mental health? *Behavior Modification*, **34**, 503–19.

Fleming S and Robinson PJ (1991) The application of cognitive therapy to the bereaved. In: Vallis TM, Howes JL and Miller PC, eds. *The Challenge of Cognitive Therapy: applications to nontraditional populations*. New York: Springer.

Fobair P *et al* (1986) Psychosocial problems among survivors of Hodgkin's disease. *Journal of Clinical Oncology*, **4**, 805–14.

Folkman S (1997) Positive psychological states and coping with severe stress. *Social Science and Medicine*, **45**, 1207–21.

Folkman S and Greer S (2000) Promoting psychological well-being in the face of serious illness: when theory, research and practice inform each other. *Psycho-Oncology*, **9**, 11–19.

Ford MF *et al* (1990) Is group psychotherapy feasible for oncology outpatient attenders on the basis of psychological morbidity? *British Journal of Cancer*, **62**, 624–6.

Fox BH (1998a) A hypothesis about Spiegel *et al.*'s 1989 paper on psychosocial intervention and breast cancer survival. *Psycho-Oncology*, **7**, 361–70.

Fox BH (1998b) Rejoinder to Spiegel *et al. Psycho-Oncology*, **7**, 518–19.

Fox BH (1999) Clarification regarding comments about a hypothesis. *Psycho-Oncology*, **8**, 366–7.

Frank JD (1971) Therapeutic factors in psychotherapy. *American Journal of Psychotherapy*, **25**, 350–61.

Freedman TG (1994) Social and cultural dimensions of hair loss in women treated for breast cancer. *Cancer Nursing*, **17**, 334–41.

Freud S (1953) Thoughts for the time on war and death (ii). In: Strachey J, ed. *Standard Edition of the Complete Psychological Works of Sigmund Freud. Volume XIV*, p. 289. London: Hogarth.

Fuller S and Swenson CH (1993) Marital quality and quality of life among cancer patients and their spouses. *Journal of Psychosocial Oncology*, **10**, 41–56.

Gil KM *et al* (2006) Benefits of the uncertainty management intervention for African American and White older breast cancer survivors: 20-month outcomes. *International Journal of Behavioral Medicine*, **13**, 286–94.

Girgis A and Sanson-Fisher RW (1998) Breaking bad news. 1: Current best advice for clinicians. *Behavioral Medicine*, **24**, 53–9.

Goedendorp MM, Gielissen MF, Verhagen CA and Bleijenberg G (2009) Psychosocial interventions for reducing fatigue during cancer treatment in adults. *Cochrane Database of Systematic Reviews*, CD006953.

Gold DB and Wegner DM (1995) Origins of ruminative thought: trauma, incompleteness, nondisclosure, and suppression. *Journal of Applied Social Psychology*, **25**, 1245–61.

Goodkin K, Antoni MH and Blaney PH (1986) Stress and hopelessness in the promotion of cervical intraepithelial neoplasia to invasive squamous cell carcinoma of the cervix. *Journal of Psychosomatic Research*, **30**, 67–76.

Goodwin PJ *et al* (1996) Randomized trial of group psychosocial support in metastatic breast cancer: the BEST (Breast Expressive-Supportive Therapy) study. *Cancer Treatment Reviews*, **22 (Suppl. A)**, 91–6.

Goodwin PJ, Pritchard KI and Spiegel D (1999) The Fox guarding the clinical trial: internal vs. external validity in randomized studies. *Psycho-Oncology*, **8**, 275.

Grandi S, Fava GA, Cunsolo A and Ranieri M (1987) Major depression associated with mastectomy. *Medical Science Research*, **15**, 283–4.

Grayling AC (2002). Death. In: *The Meaning of Things*, pp. 29–33. London: Phoenix.

Greenberg DB, Sawicka J, Eisenthal S and Ross D (1992) Fatigue syndrome due to localized radiation. *Journal of Pain and Symptom Management*, **7**, 38–45.

Greenberg LS and Safran JD (1987) *Emotion in Psychotherapy*. New York: Guilford Press.

Greer S (1985) Cancer: psychiatric aspects. In: Granville-Grossman K, ed. *Recent Advances in Clinical Psychiatry*. Edinburgh: Churchill-Livingstone.

Greer S (1995) The psychological toll of cancer. In: Horwich A, ed. *Oncology*, pp. 189–98. London: Chapman and Hall.

Greer S (1999) Mind-body research in psychooncology. *Advances in Mind-Body Medicine*, **15**, 236–44.

Greer S (2010) Bereavement care: some clinical observations. *Psycho-Oncology*, **19**, 1156–60.

Greer S and Burgess C (1987) A self-esteem measure for patients with cancer. *Psychology and Health*, **1**, 327–40.

Greer S and Watson M (1987) Mental adjustment to cancer: its measurement and prognostic importance. *Cancer Surveys*, **6**, 439–53.

Greer S, Morris T, Pettingale KW and Haybittle JL (1990) Psychological response to breast cancer and 15-year outcome. *Lancet*, **i**, 49–50.

Greer S *et al* (1992) Adjuvant psychological therapy for patients with cancer: a prospective randomised trial. *British Medical Journal*, **304**, 675–80.

Harcourt D and Rumsey N (2001) Psychological aspects of breast reconstruction: a review of the literature. *Journal of Advanced Nursing*, **35**, 477–87.

Harcourt D *et al* (2003) The psychological effect of mastectomy with or without breast reconstruction: a prospective, multicenter study. *Plastic and Reconstructive Surgery*, **111**, 1060–68.

Harrison J *et al* (1994) Concerns, confiding and psychiatric disorder in newly diagnosed cancer patients: a descriptive study. *Psycho-Oncology*, **3**, 173–9.

Heim E, Valach L and Schaffner L (1997) Coping and psychological adaptation: longitudinal effects over time and stages in breast cancer. *Psychosomatic Medicine*, **59**, 408–18.

Heinrich RL and Schag CC (1985) Stress and activity management: group treatment for cancer patients and spouses. *Journal of Consulting and Clinical Psychology*, **53**, 439–46.

Helgeson VS and Taylor SE (1993) Social comparisons and adjustment among cardiac patients. *Journal of Applied Social Psychology*, **23**, 1171–95.

Helgeson VS and Cohen S (1996) Social support and adjustment to cancer: reconciling descriptive, correlational, and intervention research. *Health Psychology*, **15**, 135–48.

Hilton BA (1994) Family communication patterns in coping with early breast cancer. *Western Journal of Nursing Research*, **16**, 366–88.

Hinton J (1967). *Dying*. London: Penguin.

Hinton J (1994) Which patients with terminal cancer are admitted from home care? *Palliative Medicine*, **8**, 197–210.

Hislop GT *et al* (1987) The prognostic significance of psychosocial factors in women with breast cancer. *Journal of Chronic Diseases*, **40**, 729–35.

Hofmana M *et al* (2007) Cancer-related fatigue: the scale of the problem. *Oncologist*, **12**, 4–10.

Holland JC and Marchini IA (1998) International psycho-oncology. In: Holland JC, ed. *Psycho-Oncology*, pp. 1165–9. New York: Oxford University Press.

Holland JC *et al* (1986) Psychosocial factors and disease-free survival in stage II breast carcinoma. *Proceedings of the American Society of Clinical Oncology*, **5**, 237 (abstract).

Hopko DR *et al* (2005) Behavior therapy for depressed cancer patients in primary care. *Psychotherapy: Theory, Research, Practice, Training*, **42**, 236–43.

Horowitz M (1986) Stress-response syndromes: a review of posttraumatic and adjustment disorders. *Hospital and Community Psychiatry*, **37**, 241–9.

Horwich A (1995) Testicular cancer. In: Horwich A, ed. *Oncology*, pp. 485–98. London: Chapman and Hall.

Hughes JE (1985) Depressive illness and lung cancer. II. Follow-up of inoperable patients. *European Journal of Surgical Oncology*, **11**, 21–4.

Hughes JE (1987) Psychological and social consequences of cancer. *Cancer Surveys*, **6**, 455–75.

Ilnyckyj A, Farber J, Cheang MC and Weinerman BF (1994) A randomized controlled trial of psychotherapeutic intervention in cancer patients. *Annals of the Royal College of Physicians and Surgeons of Canada*, **27**, 93–6.

Irvine D *et al* (1991) Psychosocial adjustment of women with breast cancer. *Cancer*, **67**, 1097–117.

Irving LM, Snyder CR and Crowson JJ (1998) Hope and coping with cancer by college women. *Journal of Personality*, **66**, 195–214.

Jacobson NS *et al* (2000) Integrative behavioral couple therapy: an acceptance-based, promising new treatment for couple discord. *Journal of Consulting and Clinical Psychology*, **68**, 351–5.

Jamison RN, Burnish TG and Wallston KA (1987) Psychogenic factors in predicting survival of breast cancer patients. *Journal of Clinical Oncology*, **5**, 768–72.

Janoff-Bulman R (1992) *Shattered Assumptions: towards a new psychology of trauma*. New York: Free Press.

Janoff-Bulman R (1999) Rebuilding shattered assumptions after traumatic life events: coping processes and outcomes. In: Snyder CR, ed. *Coping: the psychology of what works*, pp. 305–23. New York: Oxford University Press.

Jensen MR (1987) Psychobiological factors predicting the course of cancer. *Journal of Personality*, **55**, 329–42.

Jensen PT *et al* (2004) Early-stage cervical carcinoma, radical hysterectomy, and sexual function: a longitudinal study. *Cancer*, **100**, 96–106.

Johnson J (1982) The effects of a patient education course on patients with a chronic illness. *Cancer Nurse*, April issue, 117–23.

Johnson JG *et al* (2006) Development and validation of an instrument for the assessment of dependency among bereaved persons. *Journal of.Psychopathological Behavioral. Assessment*, **28**, 263–72.

Kabat-Zinn J (1990) *Full Catastrophe Living*. New York: Delacourte Press.

Kabat-Zinn J (2003) Mindfulness-based interventions in context: past, present and future. *Clinical Psychology: Science and Practice*, **10**, 144–56.

Kabat-Zinn J, Lipworth L and Burney R (1985) The clinical use of mindfulness meditation for the self-regulation of chronic pain. *Journal of Behavioral Medicine*, **8**, 163–90.

Kabat-Zinn J, Massion AO, Kristeller J *et al* (1992) Effectiveness of a meditation-based stress reduction program in the treatment of anxiety disorders. *American Journal of Psychiatry*, **149**, 936–43.

Kangas M, Bovjberg DH and Montgomery GH (2008) Cancer-related fatigue: a systematic and meta-analytic review of non-pharmacological therapies for cancer patients. *Psychological Bulletin*, **34**, 700–41.

Kausar R and Akram M (1998) Cognitive appraisal and coping of patients with terminal versus non-terminal diseases. *Journal of Behavioural Sciences*, **9**, 13–28.

Kim J *et al* (2010) The roles of social support and coping strategies in predicting breast cancer patients' emotional well-being: testing mediation and moderation models. *Journal of Health Psychology*, 15, 543–52.

Kim Y and Morrow GR (2007) The effects of family support, anxiety, and post-treatment nausea on the development of anticipatory nausea: a latent growth model. *Journal of Pain and Symptom Management*, **34**, 265–76.

Kingdon DG and Turkington D (2005) *Cognitive Therapy of Schizophrenia*. New York: Guilford Press.

Kissane DW *et al* (1997) Cognitive-existential group therapy for patients with primary breast cancer – techniques and themes. *Psycho-Oncology*, **6**, 25–33.

Kissane DW *et al* (2003) Cognitive-existential group psychotherapy for women with primary breast cancer: a randomised controlled trial. *Psycho-Oncology*, **12**, 532–46.

Kissane DW *et al* (2007) Supportive-expressive group therapy for women with metastatic breast cancer: survival and psychosocial outcome from a randomized controlled trial. *Psycho-Oncology*, **16**, 277–86.

Kornblith AB, Anderson J and Cella DF (1992) Hodgkin disease survivors at increased risk for problems in psychosocial adaptation. *Cancer*, **70**, 2214–24.

Kovacs M and Beck AT (1978) Maladaptive cognitive structures in depression. *American Journal of Psychiatry*, **135**, 525–33.

Kraemer HC, Kuchler T and Spiegel D (2009) Use and misuse of the Consolidated Standards of Reporting Trials (CONSORT) guidelines to assess research findings: comment on Coyne, Stefanek and Palmer (2007). *Psychological Bulletin*, **135**, 173–8.

Kuchler T, Bestmann B and Rappat S (2007) Impact of psychotherapeutic support for patients with gastrointestinal cancer undergoing surgery: 10-year survival results of a randomized trial. *Journal of Clinical Oncology*, **25**, 2702–8.

Kuipers E *et al* (1997) London-East Anglia randomised controlled trial of cognitive behavioural therapy for psychosis. I: Effects of the treatment phase. *British Journal of Psychiatry*, **171**, 319–27.

Ladouceur R, Gosselin P and Dugas MJ (2000) Experimental manipulation of intolerance of uncertainty: a study of a theoretical model of worry. *Behaviour Research and Therapy*, **38**, 933–41.

Lakein A (1973) *How to Get Control of Your Time and Your Life*. New York: New American Library.

Lannen PK *et al* (2008) Unresolved grief in a national sample of bereaved parents: impaired mental and physical health 4 to 9 years later. *Journal of Clinical Oncology*, **26**, 5870–76.

Larue F, Colleau S, Brasseur L and Cleeland C (1995) Multicentre study of cancer pain and its treatment in France. *British Medical Journal*, **310**, 1034–7.

Lawrence DP *et al* (2004) Evidence report on the occurrence, assessment, and treatment of fatigue in cancer patients. *Journal of the National Cancer Institute Monographs*, **32**, 40–50.

Lazarus RS and Folkman S (1984) *Stress, Appraisal and Coping*. New York: Springer.

Lee JK, Orsillo SM, Roemer L and Allen LB (2010) Distress and avoidance in generalized anxiety disorder: exploring the relationships with intolerance of uncertainty and worry. *Cognitive Behaviour Therapy*, **39**, 26–136.

Lee V *et al* (2006) Meaning-making intervention during breast or colorectal cancer treatment improves self-esteem, optimism and self-efficacy. *Social Science and Medicine*, **62**, 1133–45.

Lengacher CA, Johnson-Marland V and Post-White J (2009) Randomised controlled trial of mindfulness-based stress reduction (MBSR) for survivors of breast cancer. *Psycho-Oncology*, **18**, 1261–70.

Lepore SJ and Coyne JC (2006) Psychological interventions for distress in cancer patients: a review of reviews. *Annals of Behavioral Medicine*, **32**, 85–92.

Levine PM, Silberfarb PM and Lipowski ZJ (1978) Mental disorders in cancer patients. A study of 100 psychiatric referrals. *Cancer*, **42**, 1385–91.

Levy SM, Lee J, Bagley C and Lippman M (1988) Survival hazards analysis in first recurrent breast cancer patients: seven-year follow-up. *Psychosomatic Medicine*, **50**, 520–28.

Lewis A (1958) Between guesswork and certainty in psychiatry. *Lancet*, **i,** 171–5, 227–30.

Lewis WA and Bucher AM (1992) Anger, catharsis, the reformulated frustration-aggression hypothesis, and health consequences. *Psychotherapy*, **29**, 385–92.

Li J *et al* (2003) Mortality in parents after death of a child in Denmark: a nationwide follow-up study. *Lancet*, **361**, 363–7.

Lichtman RR and Taylor SE (1986) Close relationships and the female cancer patient. In: Andersen BL, ed. *Women with Cancer*, pp. 233–56. New York: Springer.

Lichtman RR *et al* (1985) Relations with children after breast cancer: the mother-daughter relationship at risk. *Journal of Psychosocial Oncology*, **2**, 1–19.

Link LB, Robbins L, Mancuso CA and Charlson ME (2004) How do cancer patients who try to take control of their disease differ from those who do not? *European Journal of Cancer Care*, **13**, 219–26.

Linn MW, Linn BS and Harris R (1982) Effects of counselling for late stage cancer patients. *Cancer*, **49**, 1048–55.

Llewellyn CD, Weinman J, McGurk M and Humphris G (2008) Can we predict which head and neck cancer survivors develop fears of recurrence? *Journal of Psychosomatic Research*, **65**, 525–32.

Lloyd GG (1979) Psychological stress and coping mechanisms in patients with cancer. In: Stoll BA, ed. *Mind and Cancer Prognosis*, pp. 47–59. Chichester: John Wiley & Sons.

Lloyd-Williams M and Friedman T (1999) Depression in terminally ill patients. *American Journal of Hospice Palliative Care*, **16**, 704.

Lo C *et al* (2010) Longitudinal study of depressive symptoms in patients with metastatic gastrointestinal and lung cancer. *Journal of Clinical Oncology*, **28**, 3084–9.

Low CA, Stanton AL, Bower JE and Gyllenhammer L (2010) A randomized controlled trial of emotionally expressive writing for women with metastatic breast cancer. *Health Psychology*, **29**, 460–66.

Lumley MA, Kelley JE and Leissen JCC (1997) Health effects of emotional disclosure in rheumatoid arthritis patients. *Health Psychology*, **16**, 331–40.

Lundin T (1984) Morbidity following sudden and unexpected bereavement. *British Journal of Psychiatry*, 144, 84–8.

Maciejewski PK, Zhang B, Block SD and Prigerson HG (2007) An empirical examination of the stage theory of grief. *Journal of the American Medical Association*, 297, 716–23.

McIntosh J (1974) Process of communication, information seeking and control associated with cancer. *Social Science.and Medicine*, 8, 167–87.

McLean LM, Jones JM, Rydall AC *et al* (2008) A couples intervention for patients facing advanced cancer and their spouse caregivers: outcomes of a pilot study. *Psycho-Oncology*, 17, 1152–6.

McNair D, Lorr M and Droppleman L (1971) *Manual for Profile of Mood States*. San Diego, CA: Education and Industrial Testing Service.

Magee B (1997) *Confessions of a Philosopher*. London: Weidenfeld and Nicholson.

Maguire GP, Lee EG, Bevington DJ *et al* (1978) Psychiatric problems in the first year after mastectomy. *British Medical Journal*, 1, 963–5.

Maguire P (1979) The will to live in the cancer patient. In: Stoll BA, ed. *Mind and Cancer Prognosis*, pp. 169–82. Chichester: John Wiley & Sons.

Manne SL *et al* (2005) Couple-focused group intervention for women with early stage breast cancer. *Journal of.Consulting and Clinical Psychology*, 73, 634–6.

Mannix K *et al* (2006) Effectiveness of brief training in cognitive behaviour therapy techniques for palliative care practitioners. *Palliative Medicine*, 20, 579–84.

Masters WH and Johnson VE (1970) *Human Sexual Inadequacy*. Boston, MA: Little, Brown and Company.

Mawson D, Marks I, Ramm L and Stern R (1981) Guided mourning for morbid grief: a controlled study. *British Journal of Psychiatry*, 138, 185–93.

Meichenbaum D (1977) *Cognitive-Behavior Modification: an integrative approach*. New York: Plenum Press.

Meichenbaum D (1985) *Stress Inoculation Training*. Oxford: Pergamon Press.

Mellon S, Northouse LL and Weiss LK (2006) A population-based study of the quality of life of cancer survivors and their family caregivers. *Cancer Nursing*, 29, 120–31.

Meyer TJ and Mark MM (1995) Effects of psychosocial interventions with adult cancer patients: a meta-analysis of randomized experiments. *Health Psychology*, 14, 101–8.

Middelboe T, Ovesen L, Mortensen E and Lykke BP (1995) The relationship between self-reported general health and observed depression and anxiety in cancer patients during chemotherapy. *Nordic Journal of Psychiatry*, 49, 25–31.

Mishel MH *et al* (2005) Benefits from an uncertainty management intervention for African-American and Caucasian older long-term breast cancer survivors. *Psycho-Oncology*, 14, 962–78.

Mitchell GW and Glicksman AS (1977) Cancer patients: knowledge and attitudes. *Cancer*, 40, 61–6.

Montel S (2010) Fear of recurrence: a case report of a woman breast cancer survivor with GAD treated successfully by CBT. *Clinical Psychology and Psychotherapy*, 17, 346–53.

Montgomery C, Lydon A and Lloyd K (1999) Psychological distress among cancer patients and informed consent. *Journal of Psychosomatic Research*, 46, 241–5.

Montgomery GH and Bovbjerg DH (2001) Specific response expectancies predict anticipatory nausea during chemotherapy for breast cancer. *Journal of Consulting and Clinical Psychology*, **69**, 831–5.

Moorey S (1996) When bad things happen to rational people: cognitive therapy in adverse life situations. In: Salkovskis P, ed. *Frontiers of Cognitive Therapy*, pp. 450–69. New York: Guilford Press.

Moorey S (2007) Breast cancer and body image. In: Nasser M, Baistow K and Treasure J, eds. *The Female Body in Mind: the interface between the female body and mental health*, pp. 72–89. Hove: Routledge.

Moorey S (2010) Cognitive behaviour therapy and psychoanalysis. In: Lemma A and Patrick M, eds. *Off the Couch: contemporary psychoanalytic applications*, pp. 194–211. Hove: Routledge.

Moorey S (2011) Socratic methods in adversity. In: Padesky CA and Kennerley H, eds. *Oxford Guide to Socratic Methods in CBT*, pp. 000–000. Oxford: Oxford University Press.

Moorey S and Greer S (1989) *Psychological Therapy for Patients with Cancer*. Oxford: Heinemann.

Moorey S and Greer S (2002) *Cognitive Behaviour Therapy for People with Cancer*. Oxford: Oxford University Press.

Moorey S *et al* (1991) The factor structure and factor stability of the Hospital Anxiety and Depression Scale in patients with cancer. *British Journal of Psychiatry*, **158**, 255–9.

Moorey S *et al* (1994) Adjuvant psychological therapy for patients with cancer: outcome at one year. *Psycho-Oncology*, **3**, 39–46.

Moorey S, Greer S, Bliss J and Law M (1998) A comparison of adjuvant psychological therapy and supportive counselling in patients with cancer. *Psycho-Oncology*, **7**, 218–28.

Moorey S, Frampton M and Greer S (2003) The Cancer Coping Questionnaire: a self-rating scale for measuring the impact of adjuvant psychological therapy on coping behaviour. *Psycho-Oncology*, **12**, 331–44.

Moorey S *et al* (2009) A cluster randomized controlled trial of cognitive behaviour therapy for common mental disorders in patients with advanced cancer. *Psychological Medicine*, **39**, 713–23.

Morgenthaler T *et al* (2006) Practice parameters for the psychological and behavioral treatment of insomnia: an update. An American Academy of Sleep Medicine report. *Sleep*, **29**, 1415–19.

Morize V, Nguyen DT, Lorente C and Desfosses G (1999) Descriptive epidemiological survey on a given day in all palliative care patients hospitalized in a French university hospital. *Palliative Medicine*, **13**, 105–17.

Morris T, Greer HS and White P (1977) Psychological and social adjustment to mastectomy: a two-year follow-up study. *Cancer*, **77**, 2381–7.

Morris T, Blake S and Buckley M (1985) Development of a method for rating cognitive responses to a diagnosis of cancer. *Social Science and Medicine*, **20**, 795–802.

Morris T, Pettingale K and Haybittle J (1992) Psychological response to cancer diagnosis and disease outcome in patients with breast cancer and lymphoma. *Psycho-Oncology*, **1**, 105–14.

Morrow GR (1984) Clinical characteristics associated with the development of anticipatory nausea and vomiting in cancer patients undergoing chemotherapy treatment. *Journal of Clinical Oncology*, **2**, 1170–76.

Morrow GR, Lindke J and Black PM (1991) Predicting development of anticipatory emesis in cancer patients: prospective examination of eight characteristics. *Journal of Pain and Symptom Management*, **6**, 215–23.

Morrow GR *et al* (1992) Comparing the effectiveness of behavioral treatment for chemotherapy-induced nausea and vomiting when administered by oncologists, oncology nurses, and clinical psychologists. *Health Psychology*, **11**, 250–56.

Moynihan C (1987) Testicular cancer: the psychosocial problems of patients and their relatives. *Cancer Surveys*, **6**, 477–510.

Moynihan C *et al* (1998) Evaluation of adjuvant psychological therapy in patients with testicular cancer: a randomised trial. *British Medical Journal*, **316**, 429–35.

National Institute for Clinical Excellence (2004) *Improving Supportive and Palliative Care for Adults with Cancer: the manual*. London: National Institute for Clinical Excellence.

National Institute for Health and Clinical Excellence (2009) *The Treatment and Management of Depression in Adults with Chronic Physical Health Problems. CG91*. London: National Institute for Health and Clinical Excellence.

Neimeyer RA (2006) Making meaning in the midst of loss. *Grief Matters: the Australian Journal of Grief and Bereavement*, **9**, 62–5.

Northouse LL, Dorris G and Charron-Moore C (1996) Factors affectings couples' adjustment to recurrent breast cancer. *Social Science and Medicine*, **41**, 69–76.

Northouse LL, Templin T, Mood D and Oberst M (1998) Couples' adjustment to breast cancer and benign breast disease: a longitudinal analysis. *Psycho-Oncology*, **7**, 37–48.

Novaco RW (1976) The functions and regulation of the arousal of anger. *American Journal of Psychiatry*, **133**, 1124–8.

Novaco RW (1995) Clinical problems of anger and its assessment and regulation through a stress coping skills approach. In: O'Donohue W and Krasner L, eds. *Handbook of Psychological Skills Training: clinical techniques and applications*, pp. 320–38. Boston, MA: Allyn and Bacon.

Novaco RW and Chemtob CM (1998) Anger and trauma: conceptualization, assessment, and treatment. In: Follette VM, Ruzek JI and Abueg FR, eds. *Cognitive-Behavioral Therapies for Trauma*, pp. 162–90. New York: Guilford Press.

O'Brien CW and Moorey S (2010) Outlook and adaptation in advanced cancer: a systematic review. *Psycho-Oncology*, **19**, 1239–49.

Oken D (1961) What to tell cancer patients: a study of medical attitudes. *Journal of the American Medical Association*, **175**, 1120–28.

Osborne RH *et al* (1999) The Mental Adjustment to Cancer (MAC) scale: replication and refinement in 632 breast cancer patients. *Psychological Medicine*, **29**, 1335–45.

Parkes CM (1986) *Bereavement: studies of grief in adult life*. London: Penguin Books.

Parle M, Maguire P and Heaven C (1997) The development of a training model to improve health professionals' skills, self-efficacy and outcome expectancies when communicating with cancer patients. *Social Science and Medicine*, **44**, 231–40.

Parloff MB, Waskow IE and Wolfe BE (1978) Research on therapist variables in relation to process and outcome. In: Garfield SL and Bergin A, eds. *Handbook of Psychotherapy and Behavior Change: an empirical analysis*, **2nd** edn, pp. 233–82. New York: John Wiley & Sons.

Peck A (1972) Emotional reactions to having cancer. *American Journal of Roentgenology, Radium Therapy and Nuclear Medicine*, **114**, 591–9.

Perloff LS (1983) Perceptions of vulnerability to victimisation. *Journal of Social Issues*, **39**, 41–61.

Perloff LS (1987) Social comparison and illusions of invulnerability to negative life events. In: Snyder CR and Ford CE, eds. *Coping with Negative Life Events: clinical and social psychological perspectives*, pp. 217–42. New York: Plenum Press.

Persons JB, Davidson J and Tompkins MA (2001) *Essential Components of Cognitive-Behavior Therapy for Depression*. Washington, DC: American Psychological Association.

Pettingale KW, Philalethis A, Tee DEH and Greer HS (1981) The biological correlates of psychological responses to cancer. *Journal of Psychosomatic Research*, **25**, 453–8.

Pettingale KW, Burgess C and Greer S (1988) Psychological response to cancer diagnosis. I. Correlations with prognostic variables. *Journal of Psychosomatic Research*, **32**, 255–61.

Phillips DP and Smith DG (1990) Postponement of death until symbolically meaningful occasions. *Journal of the American Medical Association*, **263**, 1947–51.

Pistrang N and Barker C (1995) The partner relationship in psychological response to breast cancer. *Social Science and Medicine*, **40**, 789–97.

Portenoy R (1989) Cancer pain. Epidemiology and symptoms. *Cancer*, **63 (Suppl. 11)**, 2298–307.

Potosky AL *et al* (2005) 5-year urinary and sexual outcomes after radical prostatectomy: results from the prostate cancer outcomes study. *Journal of Urology*, **173**, 1701–5.

Prigerson HG, Vanderwerker LC and Maciejewski PK (2008) A case for inclusion of prolonged grief disorder in DSM-V. In: Stroebe M, Hansson R, Schut H and Stroebe W, eds. *Handbook of Bereavement Research and Practice: 21st century perspectives*, pp. 165–86. Washington, DC: American Psychological Association.

Prigerson H *et al* (2009) Prolonged grief disorder: psychometric validation of criteria proposed for DMS-V and ICD-11. *PLOS Medicine,* **6(8)**, e100121.

Rabkin JG *et al* (2009) Depression, distress and positive mood in late-stage cancer: a longitudinal study. *Psycho-Oncology*, **18**, 79–86.

Raphael B (1984) *The Anatomy of Bereavement: a handbook for the caring professions*. London: Hutchinson.

Ratcliffe MA, Dawson AA and Walker LG (1995) Eysenck Personality Inventory l-scores in patients with Hodgkin's disease and non-Hodgkin's lymphoma. *Psycho-Oncology*, **4**, 39–45.

Renneker RE (1982) Cancer and psychotherapy. In: Goldberg JG, ed. *Psychotherapeutic Treatment of Cancer Patients*, pp. 000–000. New York: Free Press.

Richardson JL, Shelton DR, Krailo M and Levine AM (1990) The effect of compliance with treatment on survival among patients with hematologic malignancies. *Journal of Clinical Oncology*, **8**, 356–64.

Rieker PP, Edbril SD and Garnick MB (1985) Curative testis cancer therapy: psychosocial sequelae. *Journal of Clinical Oncology*, **3**, 1117–26.

Ringdal GI (1995) Correlates of hopelessness in cancer patients. *Journal of Psychosocial Oncology*, **13**, 47–66.

Robb KA, Williams JE, Duvivier V and Newham DJ (2006) A pain management program for chronic cancer-treatment-related pain: a preliminary study. *Journal of Pain*, **7**, 82–90.

Rodrigue JR and Park TL (1996) General and illness-specific adjustment to cancer: relationship to marital status and marital quality. *Journal of Psychosomatic Research*, **40**, 29–36.

Roesch SC *et al* (2005) Coping with prostate cancer: a meta-analytic review. *Journal of Behavioural Medicine*, **28**, 281–93.

Rosenblatt PC (2000) Parents talking in the present tense about their dead child. *Bereavement Care*, **18**, 35–8.

Ross L *et al* (2009) No effect on survival of home psychosocial intervention in a randomized study of Danish colorectal cancer patients. *Psycho-Oncology*, **18**, 875–85.

Sage N, Sowden M and Chorlton E (2008) *CBT for Chronic Illness and Palliative Care: a workbook and toolkit*. Chichester: John Wiley & Sons.

Salkovskis PM (1991) The importance of behaviour in the maintenance of anxiety and panic: a cognitive account. *Behavioural Psychotherapy*, **19**, 6–19.

Salkovskis PM and Warwick NMC (1986) Morbid preoccupations, health anxiety and reassurance: a cognitive-behavioural approach to hypochondriasis. *Behaviour Research and Therapy*, **24**, 597-602.

Sanders CM (1979) A comparison of adult bereavement in the death of a spouse, child, and parent. *Omega – Journal of Death and Dying*, **10**, 303–22.

Sandgren AK and McCaul KD (2007) Long-term telephone therapy outcomes for breast cancer patients. *Psycho-Oncology*, **16**, 38–47.

Sandgren AK *et al* (2000) Telephone therapy for patients with breast cancer. *Oncology Nursing Forum*, **27**, 683–8.

Savard J and Morin CM (2001) Insomnia in the context of cancer: a review of a neglected problem. *Journal of Clinical Oncology*, **19**, 895–908.

Savard J *et al* (2001) Prevalence, clinical characteristics, and risk factors for insomnia in the context of breast cancer. *Sleep*, **24**, 583–90.

Savard J *et al* (2006) Randomized clinical trial on cognitive therapy for depression in women with metastatic breast cancer: psychological and immunological effects. *Palliative and Supportive Care*, **4**, 219–37.

Schmale AH *et al* (1982) Pretreatment behaviour profiles associated with subsequent psychosocial adjustment in radiation therapy patients: a prospective study. *International Journal of Psychiatry in Medicine*, **12**, 187–95.

Schover LR (1998) Sexual dysfunction. In: Holland JC, ed. *Psycho-Oncology*, pp. 494–9. New York: Oxford University Press.

Scottish Intercollegiate Guidelines Network (2008) *Control of Pain in Adults with Cancer*. Guideline No. 106. Edinburgh: Scottish Intercollegiate Guidelines Network.

Segal ZV, Williams JMG and Teasdale JD (2002) *Mindfulness-Based Cognitive Therapy for Depression: a new approach to preventing relapse*. New York: Guilford Press.

Selawry O (1979) The individual and the median. In: Stoll BA, ed. *Mind and Cancer Prognosis*, pp. 39–43. Chichester: John Wiley & Sons.

Sellick SM and Crooks DL (1999) Depression and cancer: an appraisal of the literature for prevalence, detection, and practice guideline development for psychological interventions. *Psycho-Oncology*, **8**, 315–33.

Semple CJ, Dunwoody L, Sullivan K and Kernohan WG (2006) Patients with head and neck cancer prefer individualized cognitive behavioural therapy. *European Journal of Cancer Care*, **15**, 220–7.

Servaes P *et al* (1999) Inhibition of emotional expression in breast cancer patients. *Behavioral Medicine*, **25**, 23–7.

Shadish WR and Baldwin SA (2005) The effects of behavioral marital therapy: a meta-analysis of randomized controlled trials. *Journal of Consulting and Clinical Psychology*, **73**, 6–14.

Shear K, Frank E, Houch PR and Reynold CF (2005) Treatment of complicated grief: a randomized controlled trial. *Journal of the American Medical Association*, **293**, 2601–8.

Sheard T and Maguire P (1999) The effect of psychological interventions on anxiety and depression in cancer patients: results of two meta-analyses. *British Journal of Cancer*, **80**, 1770–80.

Sherman AC *et al* (2004) Group interventions for patients with cancer and HIV disease: Part I: Effects on psychosocial and functional outcomes at different phases of illness. *International Journal of Group Psychotherapy*, **54**, 29–82.

Sherwood P *et al* (2005) A cognitive behavioral intervention for symptom management in patients with advanced cancer. *Oncology Nursing Forum*, **32**, 1190–8.

Silberfarb PM and Greer S (1982) Psychological concomitants of cancer: clinical aspects. *American Journal of Psychotherapy*, **36**, 470–78.

Silverman GK, Johnson JG and Prigerson HG (2001) Preliminary explorations of the effects of prior trauma and loss on risk of psychiatric disorders in recently widowed people. *Israel Journal of Psychiatry and Related Sciences*, **38**, 202–15.

Simonton S and Sherman A (2000) An integrated model of group treatment for cancer patients. *International Journal of Group Psychotherapy*, **50**, 487–506.

Simonton S, Simonton OC and Creighton JC (1978) *Getting Well Again*. New York: Bantam Books.

Smith MT and Neubauer DN (2003) Cognitive behavior therapy for chronic insomnia. *Clinical Cornerstone*, **5**, 28–40.

Smith MT, Huang MI and Manber R (2005) Cognitive behavior therapy for chronic insomnia occurring within the context of medical and psychiatric disorders. *Clinical Psychology Review*, **25**, 559–92.

Speca M (1999) Rejoinder to Fox. *Psycho-Oncology*, **8**, 276.

Speice J *et al* (2000) Involving family members in cancer care: focus group considerations of patients and oncological providers. *Psycho-Oncology*, **9**, 101–12.

Spiegel D (1985) Psychosocial interventions with cancer patients. *Journal of Psychosocial Oncology*, **3**, 83–95.

Spiegel D and Spira J (1991) *Supportive-Expressive Group Therapy: a treatment manual of psychosocial intervention for women with recurrent breast cancer*. Stanford, CA: Stanford University School of Medicine.

Spiegel D, Bloom JR and Yalom ID (1981) Group support for patients with metastatic cancer. *Archives of General Psychiatry*, **38**, 527–33.

Spiegel D, Bloom JR, Kraemer HC and Gottheil E (1989) Effect of psychosocial treatment on survival of patients with metastatic breast cancer. *Lancet*, **ii**, 888–91.

Spiegel D, Kraemer HC and Bloom JR (1998) A tale of two methods: randomisation versus matching trials in clinical research. *Psycho-Oncology*, **7**, 371–5.

Spiegel D *et al* (1999) Group therapy for recently diagnosed breast cancer patients: a multicenter feasibility study. *Psycho-Oncology*, **8**, 482–3.

Spielberger CD, Gorsuch RL and Lushene RF (1970) *Manual for the State-Trait Anxiety Inventory*. Palo Alto, CA: Consulting Psychologists Press.

Spira JL (1998) Group therapies. In: Holland JC, ed. *Psycho-Oncology*, pp. 701–16. New York: Oxford University Press.

Stanton AL *et al* (2000a) Emotionally expressive coping predicts psychological and physical adjustment to breast cancer. *Journal of Consulting and Clinical Psychology*, **68**, 875–82.

Stanton AL, Kirk SB, Cameron CL and Danoff-Burg S (2000b) Coping through emotional approach: scale construction and validation. *Health Psychology*, **12**, 16–23.

Stiegelis HE *et al* (2003) Cognitive adaptation: a comparison of cancer patients and healthy references. *British Journal of Health Psychology*, **8**, 303–18.

Stroebe M, Schut H and Stroebe W (2007) Health outcomes of bereavement. *Lancet*, **370**, 1960–73.

Tarrier N and Maguire P (1984) Treatment of psychological distress following mastectomy: an initial report. *Behaviour Research and Therapy*, **22**, 81–4.

Tatrow K and Montgomery GH (2006) Cognitive behavioral therapy techniques for distress and pain in breast cancer patients: a meta-analysis. *Journal of Behavioral Medicine*, **29**, 17–27.

Taylor SE and Armor DA (1996) Positive illusions and coping with adversity. *Journal of Personality*, **64**, 873–98.

Taylor SE, Lichtman RR and Wood JV (1984) Attributions, beliefs about control and adjustment to breast cancer. *Journal of Personality and Social Psychology*, **46**, 489–502.

Taylor SE *et al* (1993) Optimism, coping, psychological distress, and high-risk sexual behavior among men at risk for acquired immunodeficiency syndrome (AIDS). *Journal of Personality and Social Psychology*, **63**, 460–73.

Taylor SE *et al* (2000) Psychological resources, positive illusions, and health. *American Psychologist*, **55**, 99–109.

Teasdale JD (1983) Change in cognition during depression – psychopathological implications: discussion paper. *Journal of the Royal Society of Medicine*, **76**, 1038–44.

Telch CF and Telch MJ (1986) Group coping skills instruction and supportive group therapy for cancer patients: a comparison of strategies. *Journal of Consulting and Clinical Psychology*, **34**, 802–8.

Temoshok L (1985) Biopsychosocial studies on cutaneous malignant melanoma: psychosocial factors associated with progression, psychophysiology and tumor-host response. *Social Science and Medicine*, **20**, 833–40.

Tennen H and Affleck G (1999) Finding benefits in adversity. In: Snyder CR, ed. *Coping: the psychology of what works*, pp. 279–304. Oxford: Oxford University Press.

Teno JM (1999) Lessons learned and not learned from the SUPPORT project. *Palliative Medicine*, **13**, 91–3.

Thomas C, Turner P and Madden F (1988) Coping and the outcome of stoma surgery. *Journal of Psychosomatic Research*, **4**, 457–67.

Thompson GN *et al* (2009) Prognostic acceptance and the well-being of patients receiving palliative care for cancer. *Journal of Clinical Oncology*, **27**, 5757–62.

Thwaites R and Bennett-Levy J (2007) Conceptualizing empathy in cognitive behaviour therapy: making the implicit explicit. *Behavioural and Cognitive Psychotherapy*, **35**, 591–612.

Tomarken A *et al* (2007) Factors of complicated grief pre-death in caregivers of cancer patients. *Psycho-Oncology*, **17**, 105–11.

Tremblay V, Savard J and Ivers H (2009) Predictors of the effect of cognitive behavioral therapy for chronic insomnia comorbid with breast cancer. *Journal of Consulting and Clinical Psychology*, **77**, 742–50.

Trillin AS (1981) Of dragons and garden peas: a cancer patient talks to doctors. *New England Journal of Medicine*, **304**, 699–701.

Tross S *et al* (1996) Psychological symptoms and disease-free and overall survival in women with stage II breast cancer. *Journal of the National Cancer Institute*, **88**, 661–7.

Turk DC and Fernandez E (1991) Pain: a cognitive-behavioural perspective. In: Watson M, ed. *Cancer Patient Care: psychosocial treatment methods*, pp. 15–44. New York: Cambridge University Press.

Turner R (1995) Principles of palliative care. In: Horwich A, ed. *Oncology*, pp. 199–211. London: Chapman and Hall.

Vachon MLS *et al* (1977) The final illness in cancer: the widow's perspective. *Canadian Medical Association Journal*, **117**, 1151–4.

van den Beuken-van Everdingen MH *et al* (2008) Concerns of former breast cancer patients about disease recurrence: a validation and prevalence study. *Psycho-Oncology*, **17**, 1137–45.

Vanderwerker LC, Jacobs SC, Parkes CM and Prigerson HG (2006) An exploration of associations between separation anxiety in childhood and complicated grief in later life. *Journal of Nervous and Mental Disease*, **194**, 121–3.

Van Doom C, Kasl SV, Beery KC and Prigerson HG (1998) The influence of marital quality and attachment styles on traumatic grief and depressive symptoms. *Journal of Nervous and Mental Disease*, **186**, 560–73.

von Eschenbach AC (1986) Sexual dysfunction following therapy for cancer of the prostate, testis and penis. In: Vaeth JM, ed. *Body Image, Self-Esteem and Sexuality in Cancer Patients*, pp. 48–55. Basel: Karger.

Van Heeringen C, Van Moffaert M and de Cuypere G (1990) Depression after surgery for breast cancer: comparison of mastectomy and lumpectomy. *Psychotherapy and Psychosomatics*, **51**, 175–9.

Vos MS and de Haes JC (2007) Denial in cancer patients: an explorative review. *Psycho-Oncology*, **16**, 12–25.

Vos PJ *et al* (2007) Effectiveness of group psychotherapy compared to social support groups in patients with primary non-metastatic breast cancer. *Journal of Psychosocial Oncology*, **25**, 37–60.

Watson M (1993) Anticipatory nausea and vomiting: broadening the scope of psychological treatments. *Supportive Care in Cancer*, **1**, 171–7.

Watson M and Marvell C (1992) Anticipatory nausea and vomiting among cancer patients: a review. *Psychology and Health*, **6**, 97–106.

Watson M and Greer S (1998) Coping and personality. In: Holland JC, ed. *Psycho-Oncology*, pp. 81–98. New York: Oxford University Press.

Watson M, Pettingale KW and Greer S (1984) Emotional control and autonomic arousal in breast cancer patients. *Journal of Psychosomatic Research*, **28**, 467–74.

Watson M *et al* (1988) Development of a questionnaire measure of adjustment to cancer: the MAC scale. *Psychological Medicine*, **18**, 203–9.

Watson M, Greer S, Pruyn J and Van den Borne B (1990) Locus of control and adjustment to cancer. *Psychological Reports*, **66**, 39–48.

Watson M *et al* (1994) The Mini-MAC: further development of the Mental Adjustment to Cancer scale. *Journal of Psychosocial Oncology*, **12**, 33–46.

Watson M *et al* (1999) Influence of psychological response on survival in breast cancer: a population-based cohort study. *Lancet*, **354**, 1331–6.

Weinstein M (1974) Allocation of subjects in medical experiments. *New England Journal of Medicine*, **291**, 1278–85.

Weinstein ND and Lachendro E (1982) Egocentrism as a source of unrealistic optimism. *Personality and Social Psychology Bulletin*, **8**, 195–200.

Weisman AD and Worden JW (1977) *Coping and Vulnerability in Cancer Patients*. Boston, MA: Massachusetts General Hospital and Harvard Medical School.

Weisman AD, Worden JW and Sobel HJ (1980) *Psychosocial Screening and Intervention with Cancer Patients. Project Omega*. Boston, MA: Harvard Medical School and Massachusetts General Hospital.

Wellisch DK *et al* (1992) Psychological functioning of daughters of breast cancer patients. Part II. Characterizing the distressed daughter of the breast cancer patient. *Psychosomatics*, **33**, 171–9.

Wells A (1997) *Cognitive Therapy of Anxiety Disorders*. Chichester: John Wiley & Sons.

Wells A (2000) *Emotional Disorders and Metacognition: innovative cognitive therapy*. Chichester: John Wiley & Sons.

White CA (2001) *Cognitive Behaviour Therapy for Chronic Medical Problems: a guide to assessment and treatment in practice*. Chichester: John Wiley & Sons.

Williams C (1997) A cognitive model of dysfunctional illness behaviour. *British Journal of Health Psychology*, **2**, 153–65.

Williams NL and Johnston D (1983) The quality of life after rectal excision for low rectal cancer. *British Journal of Surgery*, **70**, 460–62.

Willmoth MC and Botchway P (1999) Psychosexual implications of breast and gynaecologic cancer. *Cancer Investigations*, **17**, 631–6.

Winer EP *et al* (1999) Quality of life in patients surviving at least 12 months following high dose chemotherapy with autologous bone marrow support. *Psycho-Oncology*, **8**, 167–76.

Wirsching M, Druner HU and Herrman C (1975) Results of psychosocial adjustment to long-term colostomy. *Psychotherapy and Psychosomatics*, **26**, 245–56.

Wirsching M *et al* (1988) Psychosocial factors influencing health development in breast cancer and mastopathia. In: Cooper CL, ed. *Stress and Breast Cancer*, pp. 99–107. Chichester: John Wiley & Sons.

Wiser S and Goldfried MR (1998) Therapist interventions and client emotional experiencing in expert psychodynamic-interpersonal and cognitive-behavioral therapies. *Journal of Consulting and Clinical Psychology*, **66**, 634–40.

Wiser S and Arnow B (2001) Emotional experiencing: to facilitate or regulate? *Journal of Clinical Psychology*, **57**, 157–68.

Worden JW, Johnston LC and Harrison RH (1974) Survival quotient as a method of investigating psychosocial aspects of cancer survival. *Psychological Reports*, **35**, 719–26.

World Health Organization (1990) *Cancer Pain Relief and Palliative Care*. Geneva: World Health Organization.

Wortman CB and Dunkel-Schetter C (1979) Interpersonal relationships and cancer: a theoretical analysis. *Journal of Social Issues*, **35**, 120–55.

Zabora JR *et al* (1990) An efficient method for psychosocial screening of cancer patients. *Psychosomatics*, **31,** 192–6.

Zahlis EH and Lewis FM (1998) Mothers' stories of the school-age child's experience with the mother's breast cancer. *Journal of Psychosocial Oncology*, **16,** 25–43.

Zaider TI and Kissane DW (2010) Psychosocial interventions for couples and families coping with cancer. In: Holland JC *et al*, eds. *Handbook of Psycho-Oncology*, pp. 402–7. Oxford: Oxford University Press.

Zech D *et al* (1995) Validation of World Health Organization guidelines for cancer pain relief: a 10-year prospective study. *Pain*, **63,** 65–76.

Zee PC and Ancoli-Israel S (2009) Does effective management of sleep disorders reduce cancer-related fatigue? *Drugs*, **69** (Suppl. 2)**,** 29–41.

Zigmond AS and Snaith RP (1983) The Hospital Anxiety and Depression Scale. *Acta Psychiatrica Scandinavica*, **67,** 361–70.

Zucchero RA (1998) Marital adjustment of older adult couples with breast cancer, prostate cancer, and couples without cancer. *Dissertation Abstracts International: Section B: the Sciences and Engineering*, **59,** 3102.

Index